Sex and Sexuality
in Ancient Rome

Sex and Sexuality in Ancient Rome

LJ Trafford

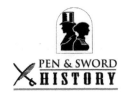

PEN & SWORD
HISTORY

First published in Great Britain in 2021 by
Pen & Sword History
An imprint of
Pen & Sword Books Ltd
Yorkshire – Philadelphia

Copyright © LJ Trafford 2021

ISBN 978 1 52678 687 6

A CIP catalogue record for this book is
available from the British Library.

Typeset by Mac Style
Printed and bound by CPI Group (UK) Ltd, Croydon, CR0 4YY

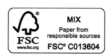

FSC
www.fsc.org
MIX
Paper from
responsible sources
FSC® C013604

Pen & Sword Books Limited incorporates the imprints of Atlas,
Archaeology, Aviation, Discovery, Family History, Fiction, History,
Maritime, Military, Military Classics, Politics, Select, Transport,
True Crime, Air World, Frontline Publishing, Leo Cooper, Remember
When, Seaforth Publishing, The Praetorian Press, Wharncliffe
Local History, Wharncliffe Transport, Wharncliffe True Crime
and White Owl.

For a complete list of Pen & Sword titles please contact

PEN & SWORD BOOKS LIMITED
47 Church Street, Barnsley, South Yorkshire, S70 2AS, England
E-mail: enquiries@pen-and-sword.co.uk
Website: www.pen-and-sword.co.uk

Or

PEN AND SWORD BOOKS
1950 Lawrence Rd, Havertown, PA 19083, USA
E-mail: Uspen-and-sword@casematepublishers.com
Website: www.penandswordbooks.com

To Kate and Clare, with gratitude for pizza, wine and gossip

Contents

List of Illustrations

1. Rome's greatest morality master, the emperor Augustus.
2. Stoic philosopher and tutor to Nero, Seneca.
3. The Tabularium on the Capitol Hill in Rome, where new citizens of the city were registered.
4. An example of a more ornate bulla Roman boys would have worn.
5. A 16th century representation of the rape of Lucretia that brought down the Roman monarchy.
6. The Vestal Virgin Tuccia being inspected while carrying water in a sieve to prove her chastity.
7. The Sleeping Hermaphroditus.
8. Terracotta statuette of a dancing youth.
9. Flavia Julia Titi, daughter of Titus.
10. Marble portrait of Matidia.
11. Julia Domna, wife to Septimius Severus, sporting her do.
12. Marble portrait of the co-emperor Lucius Verus.
13. Terracotta votive scalp, Roman, 200 BCE–200 CE.
14. A clay-baked vulva. Roman votive offering.
15. Clay-baked uterus. Roman votive offering.
16. Three Roman votive offerings: penis.
17. Marble statue of the so-called Stephanos Athlete
18. Roman surgical instruments, embryo hook and decapitator.
19. Copy of vaginal speculum, Europe, 1901–1939.
20. Statue of the roman poet Gaius Valerius Catullus in Sirmione, Lake Garda, Italy.
21. Venus and Cupid Lorenzo Lotto (Italian, Venice ca. 1480–1556 Loreto).
22. Constantine the Great, whose wife and son died in mysterious circumstances.
23. Bust in white marble of Antinous favourite of the Emperor Hadrian, worshipped in guise of Dionysius but here represented as a young man.

Introduction

There is a certain image of ancient Rome that prevails in the modern mind: one of a city soaked in depravity and decadence; a sexual free-for-all where anyone could do anything to anyone they wanted; an empire whose lack of morality was the catalyst for its decline and ultimately its fall, at least according to Edward Gibbon.

This sinful city picture is somewhat ratified by what the surviving sources and archaeological artefacts have to say: there is biographer Suetonius' frankly eye-popping account of what the Emperor Tiberius got up to on the island of Capri; the first-century CE poet Martial, whose subject matters include a rant on his girlfriend refusing to let him sodomise her, grey pubic hair, and a claim that an acquaintance is handing out dinner party invitations based solely on penis size.

Elsewhere the great unpublished can be seen expressing their sexual complaints/comments/boasts on the walls of Pompeii and Herculaneum. We are told that the gladiator Celadus makes all the girls moan, that Theophilius performs oral sex on women, and then there is the anonymous soul who believed the walls of a local villa were the perfect place to confess to his fellow townsfolk, 'I have buggered men.'

Even religion wasn't exempt from this bawdiness. The gods themselves partook in adultery, incest and even bestiality, all of which were represented in the art of the era, along with a multitude of depictions of the male sexual organ on walls, pavements, in shrines, homes, above shop doorways and on jewellery.

Naples Museum has a secret cabinet of artefacts from Pompeii and the surrounding area that were deemed too shocking to be seen by regular tourists. Visiting this secret cabinet was to be confronted with hundreds of terracotta penises, alongside frescoes of couples entwined in love making and a truly stupendous statue of the god Pan having it away with a goat.

Sex was very much on public display in ancient Rome. It was depicted in art, discussed in poetry, scrawled on walls and used in politics to smear your opponent. Is it any wonder we see ancient Rome as a 400-year-long orgy? But is this a true portrait of a society?

Rome at its height in the first century CE was home to a million people; it would be very surprising if they all held the same views on any topic, including sex and sexuality. In fact, if you dig a little deeper beneath the in-your-face depictions of penises on every street corner and explicit frescoes, the story gets a lot more complex. Despite being a society lacking the Christian notion of sexual sin, Rome was far from being a free-for-all; there were constraints, both social and legal, on sexual behaviour. In Sex and Sexuality in Ancient Rome we shall delve into these rules, looking at what was expected sexual behaviour for both men and women, and whether the reality matched the ideal. We shall look at what was understood about sex, procreation and contraception in the ancient world, examine what was truly taboo in the bedroom, and explore why there are quite so many penises depicted in Pompeii.

Leave your preconceptions at the door and let us get into bed with the Romans.

Chapter 1

Language

Those of a delicate sensibility would be wise to step away from this book now, for we are going to delve into how the ancient Romans talked about sex. Fruity is not the word, think more of a thumping great plank to the face. Words were not minced, they were hurled aggressively towards their target. But it is an important topic to start with for it helps explain much about Roman society that we will look at later, including why such extreme stories of sexual depravity attach themselves to emperors, and how female sexuality was viewed.

So, buckle up, and maybe make sure nobody is reading over your shoulder, as we take an in-depth look at how the ancient Romans talked about sex. You have been warned!

The poem begins the same as it ends, 'I will bugger you and fuck your mouths.'[1] The 'you' in question are Aurelius and Furius, whom the poet Catullus dubs as the pansy and the pervert. What had they done to inflame him so?

If you're expecting some grievous attack on a member of Catullus' family, possibly a fatal one, downgrade that expectation now. For what has upset Catullus is a criticism that his poems, which detail his great love for a woman he calls Lesbia, are unmanly.

This fucking in the mouth (in Latin, *irrumo*) is a threat tossed out by Catullus for all manner of offences. When he suspects Aurelius of having designs on a boy that he, Catullus, is seeing, he warns: 'I will get you first by fucking your mouth.'[2] He addresses to an entire tavern of men, whom he accuses of sleeping with his girl: 'Do you think I wouldn't date fuck all your mouths as you just sit there, all two hundred at once?'[3] Then there's the time he threatens the same Aurelius with having a radish and mullet fish shoved up his bum (the traditional Roman punishment for a male adulterer caught by a wronged husband – amongst other indignities).[4] All of which might lead us to conclude that Catullus is way too sensitive for his own good and should probably stay away from wine for a bit. But this extreme sexually aggressive language is not limited to Catullus' broken heart.[5] It pops up all over the place in Rome.

In 41 BCE a war broke out between Octavian, later known as the Emperor Augustus, and Mark Antony's wife, Fulvia. While Antony was out east playing with Cleopatra, Fulvia was keeping an eye on Octavian's activities in Rome and ensuring Antony's interests were taken care of. Several authors attribute the war Fulvia declared on Octavian as a tactic to entice Antony away from his Egyptian Queen lover,[6] underlining the irrationality of women, as Roman men saw it.

During this conflict the armies of Fulvia and Antony's brother, Lucius, were besieged at Perusia.[7] To break the siege Octavian's army brought in their slingshotters, these men would hurl stones at the enemy at great velocity using a length of leather that they spun around their heads before releasing. Experts have calculated that the speed these stones were projected at could reach 100 miles per hour, making them a lethally effective weapon.

Archaeologists have also found examples of slingshots with holes drilled into them, which would have caused the stones to whistle as they shot through the air. Multiply these stones by the hundreds and it must have been an unnerving sound, a further attempt at intimidating the enemy.

Eerie and unsettling whistling noise aside, there was one further tactic the Roman slingshotters used to threaten their opponents: words. Inscribed on the stones found from the siege of Perusia are some extremely barbed insults, and they come from both armies. 'Hi Octavian, you suck cock,' is the cheerful greeting on one such stone. Heading in the other direction, we find, 'I'm aiming for Fulvia's cunt.' Then there are such charming suggestions as, 'Bald Lucius Antonius and you too Fulvia, open up your arseholes,' and 'You pansy Octavian, sit on this one.'

It is quite amazing that one side of this war of filthy words will end up as Rome's great moral master, lecturing all about how good Romans should behave. For the pansy Octavian, who allegedly sucked cock and was aiming his forces directly at Fulvia's vagina, has a personality change in his thirties and emerges from a cocoon as Augustus, Rome's first emperor. One of Augustus' crusades, as we shall see later in the book, was cleaning up Roman morals and returning Rome to a golden age where young men didn't make up little ditties about married women they happened to be at war with, such as this one, which is allegedly accredited to Octavian: 'Because Antony fucks Glaphyra, Fulvia fixed this punishment for me, that I should fuck her too. That I should fuck Fulvia? What if Manius begged me to bugger him? Would I do it? Not if I had any sense.'[8]

Another source of this kind of heavy-duty insulting comes via the graffiti found at Pompeii and Herculaneum. In Pompeii alone over 11,000 different samples have been found, which give us quite an insight into the concerns of the Pompeiian town folk. There are election posters and advertisements, but also many examples like this one, 'Weep, you girls. My penis has given you up. Now it penetrates men's behinds. Goodbye, wondrous femininity!'

There are accusations that, apparently, Phileros is a eunuch, and Atimetus has got a girl up the duff. Boasts about sexual congress frequently make the walls: Apelles Mus and his brother had a good night with two girls who they both had sex with twice, we discover. Less successful was Floronius, who tells us he is with the 7th legion and that 'The women did not know of his presence. Only six women came to know, too few for such a stallion.' Poor Floronius.

Although we don't know the exact literacy figure for ancient Rome, we do know it was higher than many other time periods,[9] which does beg the question whether these pieces of graffiti were restricted to the lower (and presumably coarser) classes of the town. Not so, because some of the graffiti found is not on the outside of buildings, but rather on the inside of some very nice houses indeed. Then there is this piece from Herculaneum: 'Apollinaris, the doctor of the emperor Titus, defecated well here.' If the doctor to an emperor, a very eminent position, felt it fully acceptable and even desirable to let everyone know where he'd done a poo, I think we can safely assume that the Romans' everyday use of language might have veered to the coarse side.

As well as being coarse, to our modern sensibilities, the words used served a particular purpose. Take the example of Decimus Valerius Asiaticus, who, on being charged with effeminacy under the reign of Claudius,[10] retorted to the prosecutor, 'Ask your sons, Suillius, he said, They will confirm my masculinity.'[11] This suggests that sodomising Sullius' sons was proof against any charges of unmanly behaviour. It's not unlike that Catullus opening line we began this chapter with. It's not the words used, it's the aggressive, threatening nature of them that is very Roman.

It's hardly surprising that a city with the largest standing army in the known world, which it had used to conquer a large chunk of Europe, North Africa and the Near East, was a society that was aggressively male, and the type of insults used reflect this. Threatening sexual indignities, indeed humiliation, to your enemies was the Roman way of proving their manhood. It is worth remembering that for Roman legionaries one of the perks of sacking an enemy city was license to rape the inhabitants, be they male or female: an aggressive humiliation of the defeated city.

There was a sliding scale of insulting words, from the mild to the extremely offensive, that might be employed in any situation, be it a poem, words scrawled on a wall, a political speech, a public trial or, we must strongly assume, verbally. Insults were based on the notion of assertive and passive, of penetrating and of being penetrated. To be assertive and to penetrate was to be a man. To be passive and penetrated was to be a woman or womanish. The scale of offensiveness lay in the method of penetration, and the language reflects this.

To assert one's masculinity was to penetrate or fuck (*futuo*), this was an act solely ascribed to the male. Men could also *pedicare*, penetrate an anus. If you wanted to take the offensiveness level higher you could call another man a *cineadus* or a *catamite*, these were men who gained enjoyment through being penetrated. To be called either, therefore, was an accusation of being unmanly and effeminate. There was also an accompanying gesture to these accusations which involved scratching the head with a particular finger.

In the 50s BCE professional troublemaker Publius Clodius had a mob follow round Pompey the Great, and, acting rather like a Greek chorus, they would shout out questions such as, 'Who is a licentious imperator?', 'Who scratches his head with one finger?', and then yell their answer, 'Pompey!'[12] We are told that Pompey found this annoying, and took to hiding in his house to avoid the singing mob.[13]

There's a barbed insult from Cicero on Julius Caesar in a similar vein to the Pompey one, 'when I look at his hair, which is arranged with so much nicety, and see him scratching his head with one finger, I cannot think that this man would ever conceive of so great a crime as the overthrow of the Roman constitution.'[14] Which is a fancy way of saying Cicero didn't think Julius Caesar was man enough to make himself dictator and follow the political path he did. Irritatingly, we don't know which finger had to be used for the gesture to reach the full offensiveness level. Similarly mysterious are the continued references to the use of the left hand, which appears to suggest masturbation. A graffiti from Pompeii reads: 'When my worries oppress my body, with my left hand, I release my pent up fluids.'

The first-century CE poet Martial makes more than one reference to the left hand, noting that if his girlfriend does not turn up then his left hand helps him out in her place. He also accuses a certain Ponticus of a rather sterile love life where his left hand serves as his mistress. All of which suggests that Romans practised masturbation only with their left hand. Why the left hand? It's probably to keep the right hand free from pollution: Romans associated their right hands with noble activities such as hand shaking, signing important papers and gesticulating wildly in important political speeches.

Another body part that Romans did not want to pollute was the mouth, which they considered sacred. There were all kinds of associated reasons why: the mouth was used in religious incarnations, in politics, in oath making, and in all kinds of sacred duties. Also, a standard Roman greeting involved kissing, so you really needed to be sure where that mouth had been.

To be penetrated in the mouth was worse and far more shameful than being penetrated in the anus. It made you a *fellator*, defiling your mouth in such a fashion was viewed as particularly dirty, as hinted at in this Martial epigram: 'Zoilus, why sully the bath by bathing in it your lower extremities? It could only be made more foul, Zoilus, by your plunging your head in it.'[15]

But there was a level beneath being called a *fellator* that was even worse, the real lowest of the low. The absolute worst insult you could hurl at a Roman man was to accuse him of being a *cunus lingere*. It doesn't really need translating. It's the double whammy of insults, because not only are you defiling your mouth, you're being penetrated by the genitals of a woman. This makes you doubly passive. All of which means that the persons unknown who scrawled this on a Pompeii wall, 'Theophilus, don't perform oral sex on girls against the city wall like a dog,' really did not like Theophilus and wanted to shame him in front of the whole town. Who knows, perhaps Theophilus got his revenge and scrawled a suitably nasty retort on some other wall in that town?

Having read this far you will be unsurprised to learn that Latin has no fewer than 120 different words for penis. A *sopio* was a grotesquely oversized penis like you see on the god Priapus. At the opposite end of the scale, *pipinna* was babyish talk for the male organ, something like pee-pee.

You may have noticed that all the above insults are geared towards men, all linked to use or non-use of male appendages. But there is something else at work here and it is linked to two specific Latin words, *virtus* and *stuprum*. Both are difficult words to satisfactorily translate into English and we shall be discussing them in far greater detail later, but very roughly, *virtus* was a collection of attributes that made up the ideal Roman man and *stuprum* was a shameful act punishable by law. To commit *stuprum* was to put your *virtus* in danger. Humiliation and public shaming are the twin powers lurking in the insults and language we've looked at above.

But what of women? Were they subject to the same degree of sexually aggressive insults? The offensiveness level of Roman insults, as we have seen, is based on whether someone is behaving passively or actively in bed, based on the notion that to be a Roman male was to be dominant and active. The good Roman woman, as we shall see in a later chapter, was chaste and passive, and insults and offence directed at women tend to question these proper feminine traits. Cicero, for example, accuses the high-born Clodia of being a 'violent and impudent whore'.[16] Fulvia, who we met earlier in this chapter, behaves not as a woman ought to: 'She was a woman who took no thought for spinning or housekeeping, nor would she deign to bear sway over a man of private station, but she wished to rule a ruler and command a commander.'[17] Tacitus is clear that 'a woman, who has parted with her virtue, will not refuse other demands.'[18]

The sliding scale of insults directed at women moves from questioning their chastity to accusing them of being a literal prostitute. Once chastity has been compromised, as Tacitus comments above, then anything is possible of that woman.

I would like to apologise for the explicit content of this first chapter. I'm aware that I might have eased you into the subject more gently, but hopefully you have picked up some of the key themes and words relating to how the Romans both viewed and referred to sexual practices. We shall be returning to these ideals and ideas repeatedly as we continue on our quest to understand sex and sexuality in ancient Rome.

Chapter 2

Controlling Desire:
A Brief History of Morality Laws

After that first chapter you may be forgiven for thinking that the ancient Romans were a bunch of very potty mouthed sex obsessives. Maybe so, but there is another important element at work here and that is judgement. All those insults hurled about are designed to cast suspicion on the victim's character by the sex acts they were alleged to enjoy. Your private life is seen to be very much linked to your public life and your suitability for it.

It is here we run into an element of ancient Rome that might surprise you; it was a deeply conservative and moralistic society. There was a strong notion of what was a decent and proper way to live and successive emperors brought in laws to force the population to adhere to these standards, with admittedly mixed results. Private morals were of concern to both the state and the public, as we shall see.

Rome was a moral cesspool, that was evident to many. For the satirist Juvenal it was a city where men wore makeup, women achieved a 'happy ending' courtesy of the local masseur, schoolboys were complicit in adultery and slaves 'serviced' both master and mistress. Cato the Elder was of the firm view that the city needed a proper cleansing. Cicero was distressed that the old virtues had been so forgotten that they barely appeared in books. Pliny the Elder saw a Rome where people cultivated each other's vices rather than their good qualities. The historian Tacitus looked wistfully at the barbarian Germans and declared that 'no one there finds vice amusing or calls it up to date to seduce and be seduced.'[1]

In his introduction to his epic retelling of Rome's history, Livy was clear in what he considered the lessons of the past that he wished to pass on: 'Let him follow the decay of the national character, observing how at first it slowly sinks, then slips downward more and more rapidly, and finally begins to plunge into headlong ruin, until he reaches these days, in which we can bear neither our diseases nor their remedies.'[2]

Clearly something had gone terribly wrong with Rome, but when had this rot set in? The historian Sallust decides the rotting point was when the dictator Sulla took over Rome in the 80s BCE. Juvenal looks fondly back at the era of the Second Punic War between Rome and Hannibal. This, he decides, was a vice free era, because the men were busy fighting the Carthaginians and the women, therefore, were worn out from keeping things going in their absence. Writing a biography of the great Roman general Aemilius Paulus, Greek author Plutarch declared that this was an age 'when there were so many great and outstanding men of that glory and virtue were thick on the ground.'[3]

Interestingly, the second Punic war and the ascendency of general Aemilius Paulus both take place within the lifetime of Cato the Elder, who was convinced that *he* was living in a time of great immorality.

Clearly this golden age was one that never really existed, but Romans clung onto it and wished desperately to return to it, whether they were living like Cato in the days of the Roman republic (700 BCE to 28 BCE roughly) or under the emperors of the first and second centuries CE as Livy, Juvenal and Pliny were.

Although Romans couldn't agree when their city's descent into immorality and vice had begun, they did all agree how it had come about: because of the wealth that flooded into Rome from her empire. The philosopher Seneca muses that when men become rich they become more concerned with their appearance and obsessive about home improvements, 'how to make the walls glitter with marble that has been imported overseas, how to adorn a roof with gold, so that it may match the brightness of the inlaid floors.'[4] It's all a bit 'Grand Designs'.

In the Roman mindset there is no distinction between excesses in luxury and wealth and excesses in sex and sexual deviances. We see repeatedly in texts from the era how closely Romans associated licentious behaviour with luxury.

Cato the elder ran for the office of Censor on a platform of 'cauterising the hydra like diseases of luxury and effeminacy'.[5] The one, to Romans, led inexorably to the other. For Pliny, his contemporary's obsession with the acquiring wealth had led them to abandon the pursuit of knowledge and the begetting of children. Juvenal's view was that the desire for money had caused all to abandon sexual chastity whether they be schoolboys or brides, matrons or widows. In describing Eppia, a well brought-up lady who eloped with a gladiator, Juvenal says of her, '[she] was luxury-reared, cradled by Daddy in swansdown, brought up to frills and flounces.'[6] The luxury she has experienced had softened her towards sexual immorality.

Women were often on the receiving end of these concerns about the corrupting nature of luxury and wealth. Pliny the Elder recounts seeing the Empress Lollia Paulina, wife to Caligula, attending an ordinary banquet heaped in jewels worth 40 million sesterces. Then there is the fanciful story of Cleopatra dissolving a pearl in vinegar and drinking it in order to win a bet that her dinner would cost 10 million sesterces.

In 215 BCE an attempt was made to limit the amount of money that women could spend on themselves. The Lex Oppia restricted women to possessing no more than half an ounce of gold and forbade them from wearing overly colourful clothing. It was argued that women, 'given a free rein to their undisciplined nature, to this untamed animal, and then expect them to set a limit on their own license!'[7] The law was repealed in 195 BCE.

It wasn't just experiencing luxury that dented natural Roman morals, it was also the greed for more of the same that had warped them. The link between greed and excess was so established in the Roman mind that whenever we find laws aimed at controlling sexual behaviour, we also find sumptuary laws limiting prices or access to luxury goods. Any Roman who displayed an excessive love of luxury was bound to show similar excesses in their sexual life.

This link between luxury and sexual immorality is evident from the extreme accounts of the behaviour of some emperors. Caligula twinned his debauching of his friend's wives with spending habits so large he bankrupted the ample treasury that his predecessor, Tiberius, had left him. Nero's golden house, a building that came to display the most opulent, luxurious behaviour of the ancient world, was matched by his over-the-top antics with the palace slaves, who he co-opted into strange, sexual, role play games.

That these themes of avarice and immorality appear so often in Roman texts demonstrates just how worrying they found it. The behaviour of a citizen in the privacy of their bedroom (or elsewhere) was of deep public concern to Romans. A standard political speech inevitably accuses a rival of sexual deviance of some sort. This is perhaps best exemplified in Cicero's Second Philippic speech attacking Mark Antony, where the latter is said to have been a drunk, engaged in a same-sex relationship with his friend, Curio, become a male prostitute, dressed as a woman and consorted with actresses of low standing. Which is quite a lot to fit into the few years of youth.

Roman thinking was that dubious private behaviour meant dubious public behaviour. Someone who behaved inappropriately in the bedroom was not fit for government of the greatest city in the world. Such were the concerns around the private lives of citizens that the state got involved. Attempts were made to force Romans to comply with what was felt to be 'proper' sexual behaviours.

One weapon the state had at its disposal was the role of censor. The main task of the censors (for there were always two of them) was to keep a register of the citizen body of Rome, along with such extra details as their class and their wealth. The censor also had another quite unique power: as well as registering the members of each class, he could, if he chose to, demote them to a lower class or expel them entirely. He might do this if he felt they were lacking in the right attributes suitable to their class. Greek historian Plutarch, in his life of Cato the elder, notes that the censor's duties included regulating any departure from the traditional established way of living.

This had the greatest impact for the highest classes, the equestrians and the senators. To be either you needed money, a lot of money. The qualification for the rank of equestrian was 400,000 sesterces, for a senator one million sesterces. To put this in context, the pay for a Roman legionary, who was by no means considered poor (hence why people enlisted), was set at 1200 sesterces per year in the late first century CE.

Men from the equestrian and senatorial classes could stand for election to the public positions involved in running both the city and the empire. To serve the state in a public capacity was of great importance to Romans; it was the greatest of honours and surrounded you with a halo of prestige. It was also a good opportunity to make some serious money, particularly if you made it to becoming a provincial governor. To be expelled from the Senate was to lose your position, your influence and your power. It was also deeply shaming for you and your entire family.

It was for this position of censor that Cato the Elder stood in 184 BCE. His election campaign was quite something. Rather than encouraging people to vote for him, he instead stood on the rostra[8] and delivered threats to those he saw as not conforming to traditional standards. He promised that he, Cato, would purify the city of the stench of immorality once and for all, further declaring that only he could be trusted to do this. The people of Rome had good reason to believe Cato would deliver on his promises, for he was very much a man who lived by his words. In a city that was gaining unimaginable wealth, Cato alone appeared immune to its corrupting influence.

There is an abundance of stories relating to Cato's philosophy of a simple life: we are told that he never wore any item of clothing that cost over 100 drachma; that he was so horrified to inherit a beautifully embroidered Babylonian robe that he sold it off immediately; and that not one of the walls in his house was plastered. When he served as praetor of Sardinia, he conducted his duties visiting cities on foot with but a single assistant, hardly showing off the pomp and majesty that was Rome to the provinces.

Luxury did not interest Cato, instead hard work did. It was said that he worked the fields alongside his slaves and even dressed in the same clothes that they wore. He ate food and drank wine that was the same as the rations he gave his workers. But let us be clear that Cato certainly did not see himself as equal to his slaves, he was very much not the enlightened slave owner. He deliberately fostered discontent amongst the workforce so that they couldn't mobilise against him and happily sold off slaves once he found them no longer useful.

Cato's disinterest and dislike of luxury and the example he set in his own life made him, in voters' eyes, the perfect man for the job of protecting Rome's traditions from polluting outside influences. They duly ignored the seven other, state approved candidates for censor who promised not to upset their lives too much and voted for Cato. His moralising and grandstanding on the horrors of luxury and wealth had hit the public mood just right.

Once in power, Cato fulfilled his shouty potential by letting rip with the cleansing of the Senate, not always unjustifiably. As with all populists, Cato became popular because he'd hit upon a truth; Rome was changing quickly in ways the population wasn't always comfortable with and there was corruption present at the highest level.

One of Cato's measures was to cut off the pipes that the rich were using to direct what was public water into their homes, putting an end to the impressive fountains and water features they had been sneakily running using a purloined supply. He increased the value of items such as jewellery, furniture and posh dinnerware to discourage the accumulation of objects and to raise taxes on such luxury goods.

However, the expulsion of a politician from the Senate for the crime of embracing his wife in daylight in front of their daughter veers towards the ridiculous. For his work in prying into the lives of others, judging them for it and then doing his best to ruin it, Cato was rewarded with a statue of himself. The inscription read, 'When the Roman state was tottering to its fall, he was made censor, and by helpful guidance, wise restraints, and sound teachings, restored it again.'[9] Although clearly he didn't, because luxury, wealth, immorality and bad living are topics of just as much concern for centuries afterwards.

Fifty years after Cato's tough love approach, another censor, the impressively named Quintus Caecilius Metellus Macedonicus, in his appointment speech hit out at public morals. Macedonicus' proposal was that Rome's moral decline could only be halted by compulsory matrimony. Others disagreed and his proposal did not make it into law.

However, some form of control over public morals did make it into law in the shape of the Lex Scantinia. The Lex Scantinia is irritatingly elusive. From a few scattered references across sources we can deduce that these laws were aimed at curbing certain behaviours, but we don't have enough evidence to confidently assert what these behaviours were.

References to the Lex Scantinia pop up in relation to that slippery word, *stuprum* – a shameful act. We can make a few assertions with the information we have: *stuprum* only applied to the freeborn and the Lex Scantinia appears to have been aimed at protecting the freeborn from offences committed against them. References would seem to suggest these offences included pederasty, adultery and misbehaviour with a vestal virgin. There were likely many other acts listed, but we have no idea what they are. Although that is perhaps telling, we cannot grasp the full details of the Lex Scantinia because there are not enough references to it for us to form a full picture, which in turn shows that these laws were rarely used in prosecutions. However, the Lex Scantinia, sketchy as it is and likely rarely invoked, is important for being a state defined mechanism for dealing with acts considered morally dubious.

A century after the Quintus Caecilius Metellus Macedonicus speech it gets another airing in full by Rome's first emperor, Augustus. We met Augustus in the last chapter in his previous incarnation as Octavian, who gets accused of all manner of moral improprieties. However, Augustus is a one-man morality machine who spends his days trying to force his subjects to live properly and decently.

Augustus' efforts are the first comprehensive attempt to tackle public morals, as he boasted in the account of his achievements, the *Res Gestae*, 'Through new laws passed on my proposal I brought back many of the exemplary practises of our ancestor which had fallen into neglect.'

Augustus took it much further than expelling the odd senator for lapses in judgement, such as Cato the Elder did, instead he instituted a series of morality laws. Known as the Lex Julia and the Lex Poppaea, these offered incentives for good moral behaviour and penalties for bad, and thankfully, we have a lot more information on them than the sketchy Lex Scantinia.

Under these laws marriage and childbearing were positively encouraged. Women who produced three children were given a tax break and could throw off the imposition of a guardian. Former female slaves were offered the same, though they were expected to produce four children for the same incentives. As the minimum age for manumission from slavery was thirty, you do have to wonder how possible this was. A later amendment, the Flavian Municipal law, allowed in the case of a tied election for the candidate who was married and had produced children to be declared the winner.

Alongside the carrot was the stick: if you did not marry you could expect to be fined. This was enforced on women above the age of twenty and men aged twenty-five and over, with an upper age limit of fifty for women and sixty for men. Should a marriage end in divorce a couple were given six months' grace before they were penalised for their single status. Widowers were given a year.

Augustus also introduced harsh penalties for adultery within marriage. Rome was a patriarchal society, so unsurprisingly women got the far rawer deal. Whereas men only counted as adulterers if their partner was a freeborn married woman, women were penalised for sleeping with anyone who was not their husband.

As well as promoting marriage there was an emphasis on it being the right kind of marriage, with restrictions on who was able to marry who based on their class. Those of the senatorial class were more restricted in who they could legally marry compared with those further down the class structure. For example, the lower born freeborn were permitted to marry ex-slaves, the senatorial class were not. Those at the very bottom of the ladder had their status enshrined: all classes were forbidden from marrying actors, actresses, pimps and prostitutes. People working in these professions were known as *infames* and had many other legal and social restrictions placed upon them (which we shall delve into in a later chapter).

It's worth noting what isn't in the Lex Julia and Poppaea, as well as what is. There is no mention or restrictions on divorce and nothing whatsoever to do with same-sex relationships. Roman concerns were very different to the later Christian world.

A hundred years later there was another moral reformer in the Augustus mould, the emperor Domitian. Ruling from 81–96 CE, Domitian tightened up the adultery laws passed by Augustus, issuing harsher penalties for those convicted. Domitian took on the role of censor personally and proved himself the heir of Cato the Elder by expelling an official from the Senate because of his love of acting and dancing.

Domitian also tackled other moral issues, banning the castration of boys and restricting the price of eunuchs, so that the slave traders could not profit. The prostitution of freeborn boys was also strictly prohibited (note not slaves or ex-slaves). All of which is the subject of some fairly toe-curling poetry from court poet Martial, who exclaims breathlessly, 'Before this, Caesar, you were loved by boys, and youths, and old men; now infants also love you!'[10]

There are later tweaks in the second century CE to both adultery laws and those concerning eunuchs, extending who is liable for prosecution in connection to both offences. For adultery, the law is extended beyond the couple who are engaged in an adulterous affair to anyone who might be classed as having facilitated it by offering up their house as a location for sex.

Between the years 200 and 400 CE it is notable that the law in general gets a lot harsher. The number of crimes that are now punishable by death quadruples in this period and includes transgressions of morality.

Whereas under first-century moral masters like Augustus and Domitian you could expect to lose your status and perhaps be exiled after being prosecuted for adultery, in these later centuries you now faced execution.

The Augustan laws do not mention same-sex partners in any capacity whereas in later centuries it is overtly spelt out. Justinian, who ruled as a Christian emperor from 527 CE, talks of disgraceful lusts and acts contrary to nature. The chance to repent is offered but if refused Justinian is happy to inflict, what is stated as 'extreme punishments'.

Extreme punishments were also meted out to free women who had sexual intercourse with a slave, male prostitution, anyone in the business of creating eunuchs, rapists and anyone present when a rape occurred, amongst many other offences. Abortion, which is absent from all prior rulings on private life, now features as an offence. As with much of Roman law, the punishment here is linked to social status, a lower-class woman could expect to be sent to the mines, an upper-class woman might escape with only exile.

The fact that there are so many laws associated with the private life of citizens over so many centuries clearly shows what a real concern it was to Romans. These laws show us what was considered undesirable moral behaviour. In our next chapter we will move away from all the moaning about kids today and explore what it was that Pliny, Juvenal, Cato et al. wanted to return to. What were the attributes and behaviours that made a man the perfect Roman? And what about women: what was their standard to live up to?

Chapter 3

Ideals: The Virtuous Man

The Romans had a word for how men ought to be, *virtus*. It comes from *vir* meaning man and it is one of those words that doesn't easily translate. The English language may have co-opted *virtus* as virtue, but it was so much more than that.

Virtus was a combination of qualities that made up the perfect Roman male who could be used in service of the state. Unsurprisingly, given the Roman tendency for conquering, prowess on the battlefield was an important part of acquiring *virtus*. But it was not enough to be a good fighter, you also had to face that battle with both courage and vigour. This energy and fearlessness were expected outside of war in your public life too, alongside other characteristics such as self-control, fortitude and toughness. But also softer attributes such as clemency and prudence.

This concept of *virtus*, of trying to be the best you can, flows through the letters of stoic philosopher and tutor to Emperor Nero, Seneca. Stoicism split virtue into four aspects; wisdom, justice, courage and moderation. They maintained that happiness was obtained through adherence to these virtues.

Seneca spends an inordinate amount of words informing his correspondents how they can improve themselves for their own future happiness. This includes such tips as choosing friends wisely, living simply but not drawing attention to yourself in doing so, being kind to your slaves, not letting the thought of your imminent death upset you, and reading a lot. Reading Seneca's letters and their emphasis on sobriety, rejection of luxury and being a good person, you cannot help but reflect how little any of this rubbed off on his pupil, Nero.

The physician Galen has a practical suggestion for how to obtain that necessary *virtus*; appoint someone to follow you round and point out all your mistakes. If having someone constantly criticising your every move sounds soul destroying, it truly is. As Galen warns, 'In the early stages this will be difficult and will be accomplished only at the cost of much evident unhappiness.'[1]

History provided ample examples of *virtus*-enthused men to emulate. The examples on offer tend to date back to the Republican period, the part of Rome's history where they were starting to conquer their neighbours but had yet to be diminished morally by the flood of money and luxury those conquests brought. Is there anything we might learn from these great and outstanding men about what made the perfect Roman man?

The merciful victor: Aemilius Paullus

'A reputation arising from valour, justice, and trustworthiness. In these virtues he at once surpassed his contemporaries.' So says Greek biographer Plutarch on the Roman general Aemilius Paullus who lived between 229 BCE and 160 BCE.

Paullus demonstrates for us ample evidence of the *virtus* qualities in action. He was victorious in battle against an enemy army four times the size of his force and in the aftermath of this victory he made it clear he would be lenient with the defeated foe, the Ligurians.[2] The Ligurians, we are told, trusted Paullus and handed over their ships and settlements to him. He kept his word and restored these settlements to them, with reasonable terms of surrender, which is a nice example of success in war, clemency and oath keeping: a triple whammy of *virtus*.

This clemency is evident in his treatment of the Macedonian king, Perseus, another one of Paullus' defeated foes. After the obligatory triumph, which Perseus was forced to take part in, Paullus took pity on the former king and arranged for him to be moved to a prison where he could live out his days. Paullus here is praised for his strong desire to assist an enemy he had defeated, although given that Perseus later starved to death, I think we can confidently say Paullus' assistance and care did not spread so far.

On the personal front he is singled out for the way he stoically coped with the deaths of his two sons, the first of whom died a few days before that triumph over Perseus. When his second son died, Paullus is praised for going to the assembly that very day and addressing the people with a speech on the nature of fortune – recognising that while at the height of his public fortunes his private ones had perished.

The *virtus* of Aemilius Paullus is probably best demonstrated at his funeral where his bier was carried by a group of Spaniards, Ligurians and Macedonians. They were from nations that Paullus had personally been responsible for conquering and adding to the empire. Yet we are told they were grateful for it and that after conquering them, Paullus had continued to visit the regions and 'cared for them as if they had been members of his own household or family.'[3] This was what the Romans admired, the dual aspects of annihilating an enemy in battle yet treating them honourably afterwards.

Aemilius Paullus was the near perfect Roman to Plutarch, demonstrating all the proper virtues and behaving impeccably – with one exception. Plutarch can't bring himself to approve of Paullus divorcing his first wife, given she had produced children for him. His research can find no reason for this divorce or any wrongdoing on behalf of Paullus' wife and so he concludes, 'it is the slight, often repeated irritation of petty annoyances and incompatibilities that is responsible for irreparable estrangements in marriages.'[4] This is a conclusion reached with no actual evidence and makes you wonder if it's more a reflection of Plutarch's own marriage rather than Paullus'.

From the farm he came: Cincinnatus

Another Roman hero from the very early days of the republic who has full *virtus* on display is Lucius Quinctius Cincinnatus.[5] Cincinnatus' claim to fame is that he was made dictator of Rome twice and each time he handed back the power once he was no longer needed. There's a lesson there for Julius Caesar.

The word dictator has a very different meaning to us today than it did to the ancient Romans. The role of dictator was a position granted by the Roman Senate to a single individual to take control of the state in an emergency and for a limited time only. There were several times in the history of Rome when the appointment of a dictator was deemed necessary. We tend to find dictators appointed during times of war and upheaval, which indeed was the case with Cincinnatus.

The following tale, I'm afraid, reads like a film script. In 458 BCE Rome's neighbours, the Sabines, launched a full-on invasion, and having failed to penetrate the city walls they wreaked their frustration on the countryside, destroying crops. An army went to confront them only to find themselves under siege. Desperate times called for desperate measures, and the only man who could save Rome; enter Cincinnatus.

But where was Rome's saviour? Well, he was at that very moment working on his small three-acre farm. There is quite the tragic backstory that accounts for Cincinnatus' poverty and absence from Rome. His wayward son had been charged with numerous serious offences, including political violence and murder, and, facing a sure-fire conviction, had fled Rome in the dead of night. The state required justice and without a defendant to put on trial Cincinnatus was forced to pay for his son's sins. He lost absolutely everything, which is how he ended up living a simple life on the farm while Rome faced her greatest ever calamity.

The representatives from Rome found Cincinnatus on his farm ploughing as the sun dipped beneath the horizon. They explained that the Senate had appointed him dictator. Given Cincinnatus' tragic past he was quite within his rights to tell them to get lost. But of course, he didn't; otherwise this would not be a story of Roman *virtus*. 'He told his wife Racilia to run to their cottage and fetch his toga. The toga was brought, and wiping the grimy sweat from his hands and face he put it on.'[6] What a man!

Cincinnatus accompanied them to Rome, where he took up the position of dictator and rode out to rescue the besieged Roman army and defeat the enemy, which he did remarkably swiftly. A mere fifteen days after he accepted the powers that came with the dictatorship, he handed them back, and returned to his plough once more. Roll credits.

The second part of Cincinnatus' story takes place nineteen years later, when Rome faced another catastrophe, this time from within its own walls. A man named Spurius Maelius had been gaining popular support by distributing grain to the poor, a move that had won him several elections and propelled him ever upwards. But when he'd reached the highest position possible, that of consul, it didn't sate his ambition. He needed more: he needed to be king.

Rumours spread that Maelius was gathering arms and people for a full-on revolt against the state. In these perilous times there was only one man they could call upon, and he was out ploughing again. Or perhaps not, because in 439 BCE Cincinnatus was aged eighty, something he reminded the Senate of. But, in what would be a very rousing scene in the film, the Senate shouted down his objections and declared that he had more wisdom and courage in his heart than all of them put together.

No battle scene this time, but rather a tense interrogation scene between Cincinnatus and Maelius, which opens with the terrific line (cribbed straight from Livy again) 'the dictator requires your presence'. Maelius, it hardly needs to be said, is executed. His house is demolished, and the space where it had stood left as a permanent reminder of a plot that failed. After a bit of mopping up, Cincinnatus again handed back the powers of the dictator after a mere twenty-one days in power and then strode back to his plough.

Now you may think the key part of this story, nay this legend, is the bit about the man who'd been humiliated and humbled by the Senate being called back to help when times get tough. About how he was rehabilitated and even cheered by the very men who'd destroyed his life. But no, the element that pops up again and again in Roman literature is the part where he sets down his plough, takes up the mantle of public office and then hands it back again. This is the most Roman of actions, the very highest display of *virtus* on offer: the man who gave up power.

But also, the farm bit is important. Romans have a very strange obsession with agriculture and working the land. In the mythical golden age it is presumed that every decent Roman would have been exhausting himself in honest toil. Remember Cato the Elder working alongside his slaves? Well, he wrote an entire treatise on agriculture which tells us, with shades of Cincinnatus, that, 'it is from the farming class that the bravest men and the sturdiest soldiers come.'

The simple (but wealthy) farmer

Lucius Junius Moderatus Columella was the author of a similar work to Cato the Elder's on agriculture, and he is very clear on the link between farming and Rome's past successes. 'But, by heaven, that true stock of Romulus, practised in constant hunting and no less in toiling in the fields, was distinguished by the greatest physical strength and, hardened by the labours of peace, easily endured the hardships of war when occasion demanded, and always esteemed the common people of the country more highly than those of the city.'[7]

He has much to say, like those other writers we looked at in our second chapter, on the decadence of city life ruining the moral character of Romans, though the intended readers of Columella's volumes are not exactly working the land themselves. Columella dedicates quite a bit of time to discussing the perfect spot to build your villa, which includes a thoughtful suggestion on the positioning of your summer bedrooms and bathrooms (the plural here is telling).

Columella's farmers are also presumed to own a large body of slaves to work their land. The passages devoted to slave management contain crucial advice such as, 'I perceived that their unending toil was lightened by such friendliness on the part of the master, I would even jest with them at times and allow them also to jest more freely.'[8]

Our 'kind' slave master recommends others follow his practise of rewarding female slaves who produce a lot of offspring with an exemption from work and to carefully inspect your shackled slaves to ensure they are properly contained.

Columella's book is extremely detailed on all aspects of agriculture, covering subjects such as what makes a good slave overseer, where to position your cattle shed, soil quality and the best way to yoke oxen. Although Columella's farmer is no Cincinnatus, he is a learned man who has taken the time to understand the subject. Time that might otherwise be spent in dubious city pursuits.

Being a Roman man was to be physical, hard-working, honest and trustworthy. It was to be kind yet also harsh when required. It was to take on the yoke of responsibility to the state, but not to be greedy for power. It was to be learned and knowledgeable. All of which was pretty much a full-time job, but this was good because idleness held its own particular dangers. A certain amount of leisure was acceptable, but too much could have a catastrophic impact on your *virtus*. Never was this more in play than the period after a Roman male came of age.

Youth – the dangerous age

In childhood Roman boys wore a special amulet around their necks known as a bulla. Bullae could be a simple leather pouch or they could be an ornate gold locket, depending on your status and spending power. The bulla was a form of protection for inside each one, whether it be leather or gold, were kept protective amulets designed to keep away evil spirits and misfortune from the child.

Bullae were also a visible indicator of age, meaning hands off to any sexual advances. Freeborn boys possessed something called *pudicitia*, meaning modesty, and to violate this was to put yourself at the risk of prosecution.

At around the age of fifteen Roman boys came of age and became men. For elite Romans this would be marked by a ceremony. In the morning the boy took off his protective bulla and childhood toga, known as the toga praetexta, and put on a white tunic and the toga virilis of adulthood. A sacrifice would take place dedicated to the household gods, the Lares, and then the boy, accompanied by his family, would make their way to the Forum.

From the Forum they would walk up the Capitol Hill to the Tabularium, which was the records office for Rome and where the boy would be entered onto the register as a citizen. A trip to the Temple of Jupiter followed, where the boy would offer up the shavings from his first beard. Although few probably did so with the glorious extravagance of Nero, who placed his shavings in a golden box adorned with priceless pearls. After the beard dedication, details are sketchy on what happened next, but let us assume they probably went home and had a bit of a party.

Donning the toga virilis was an important moment in a boy's life, one filled with significance and ceremony, and one that officially marked him as a Roman man, after which this new Roman man would do, well, not a lot. Men of the elite, senatorial class were expected to pursue a public career climbing up the ladder of positions, known as the *cursus honorum*, that would take them all the way up to the highest position possible, that of consul. However, you weren't eligible for the first rung on this ladder until you had reached the age of twenty-five, which meant that there were an awful lot of young men aged fifteen to twenty-five hanging about Rome with too much money and too much time on their hands.

The poet Horace talks about how a beardless youth relieved of his teacher could find enjoyment in horses, dogs and sunbathing on the Campus Martius. Other pursuits in which the Roman youth might indulge in included wrestling, hunting, bathing, going to the theatre or the amphitheatre and gambling. In the Roman family the head, or paterfamilias, was in control of all the finances of family members, including adult sons. Although this had a downside in making adult males beholden to their fathers for an income, the upside was that the paterfamilias was also solely responsible for any family debts – which had to make gambling all the more appealing for the young, bored male.

This might all sound like a pleasant gap year before knuckling down to decades of hard work but to Roman eyes it was a uniquely dangerous time. As Horace concludes on his beardless youth, 'He is soft as wax to be seduced into vice.'[9]

Having only just stepped out of his childhood toga and shaven off that first beard, the Roman youth was seen to be vulnerable to all manner of bad influences. What happened in this period of his life could taint his reputation forever. It would certainly be thrown back in his face the moment he stood for public office or even legal cases in which he might later be involved.

Cicero, the undisputed king of raking up decades-old muck and throwing it at speed, has some advice for parents, 'Give youth some leeway then; allow our young men to stray a little; do not rein in every pleasure; let the ideal and forthright life suffer an occasional check; let reason give way now and then to appetite and desire. Provided that in all this some bounds are not overstepped.'[10] The bounds that should not be overstepped, Cicero continues, are fooling around with another man's wife, getting into debt, violence, intrigue and crime.

There is a peculiar high jink of the young Roman male that would fit Cicero's criteria of violence and crime, the practice of dressing down, going to local taverns and beating up the punters. This is a strange activity that even emperors might indulge in. Nero was said to enjoy beating up men returning from dinner and throwing them into the sewers. Nero's pal and later emperor, Otho, liked to pick on drunks, wrapping them up in a blanket and tossing them in the river. The Emperor Commodus was said to have drunk the resources of the empire dry by his evening rambles to taverns and brothels.

Mark Antony, according to Cicero, assumed his toga of manhood and then took to being a rent boy; as you do. An accusation that Antony hurls back, not at Cicero but Octavian, who he claims sold himself for 3,000 gold pieces, which could be taken as a compliment because that's a huge amount of money. Antony also claimed that Octavian was only adopted by Julius Caesar as his heir because he submitted to Caesar sexually, which is as neat a piece of ancient virtue signalling as you'll see: look at me, I wasn't Caesar's heir because I would not stoop to such gross antics; unlike him.

The message here is that not only could the Roman youth stumble into vice of their own accord, they could also be coerced into it. However, Julius Caesar is an amateur in corrupting youth compared to Lucius Sergius Catiline. Having failed to win a consular election in 64 BCE, Catiline decided instead to overthrow the Roman republic and grasp all the power for himself.

As part of this power grab plan, Catiline had been putting together an army that consisted of many young men. A fact that Cicero uses in a series of devastating speeches against this would be revolutionary. Catiline is the ultimate corrupter of youth: 'These boys, so witty and delicate, have learnt not only to love and to be loved, not only to sing and to dance, but also to brandish daggers and to administer poisons.'[11]

For Cicero, Catiline's baleful influence on these young men has taken them beyond drinking parties and prostitutes, beyond gambling debts and bankruptcy, into a wholly new criminal pastime of conspiring against the state. This was heinous indeed. Youth was truly a dangerous age.

After surviving the pitfalls and treachery of youth the fully grown Roman man then had an entire lifetime to struggle with his self-control and acquire all the attributes that made up *virtus*. This is a subject of endless writings from Cicero to Galen to Seneca to philosophers of every ilk. It was a constant struggle to get the balance just right: to live simply but not to be ungenerous to guests, to offer clemency but not to appear weak, to fight well but not to overstep the mark into cruelty. It had to be exhausting.

But where does sex feature in all this? We have seen it was important to avoid unwise liaisons with older men when passing through adolescence, but what thereafter? What kind of sex did the virtuous man partake in?

Firstly, in moderation, nothing too excessive. Secondly, with the correct type of partner, as demonstrated by this quote from a Plautus play, 'Love whatever you want, as long as you stay away from married ladies, widows, virgins, young men and free boys.'[12] Why not these people? Because they were protected under the laws of *stuprum*. Notably excluded from this list are slaves and prostitutes.

But for all the acres of papyri dedicated to discussing *virtus*, sex really doesn't feature much. Yes there is some space given to the dangers of excessive lust, but concepts such as keeping sex within marriage or abstinence are not concepts that the Romans recognise. Unless of course you are a woman, who, unlike men, had an ideal to live up to that was very much linked to how they used their body, as we shall see in the next chapter.

Chapter 4

Ideals: The Chaste Woman

Constrained lives

In the last chapter we looked at the character of the ideal Roman man, let us now consider women. Roman women, as in other historical eras, had fewer rights then men. They were severely limited in what role they could play in public life, they could not stand for public offices, they could not vote, they could not serve in the army.

In their private lives they remained under the control of a male guardian; in childhood this would be the paterfamilias. The paterfamilias had an enormous amount of control over all the members of his household, be they male, female or slave. He controlled the finances of the household members, even when they were adults, and could also dish out physical punishment for what he saw as errant or unacceptable behaviour. The father of the future emperor Otho, we are told, regularly flogged his son for his wild and extravagant behaviour, although it apparently had little effect on Otho's behaviour.

Such was the paterfamilias' control that he even had power of life or death over his household. Legally he could murder members of his family: for example, if he caught any of his womenfolk in the act of adultery he could kill both parties.[1] We have very few examples of a paterfamilias killing members of his own family, and the examples we do have date way back to the time of Romulus; a certain Egnatius Maetennus was said to have clubbed his wife to death for drinking wine, but was acquitted of her murder. Pliny the Elder tells us of another woman, who remains unnamed, who was starved to death by her family for stealing the keys to the wine cellar, but there is little in the way of corroborating evidence for this story.

One way the paterfamilias does exercise his power of life or death was after the birth of any child to his extended family. It was his decision whether the child should be reared or exposed. The exposure of babies went right back to the very founding of Rome, with twins Romulus and Remus left beside a river to die. It pops up repeatedly in mythology as a plot device, which will end in a happy familiar reunion later on. Unless you are Oedipus, whose reunion with his birth parents did not run so smoothly.[2]

In mythology there is always a handy shepherd just off screen ready to enter the story by stumbling across the exposed infant and raising them as their own prior to the proper plot kicking off. In real life, certainly on the streets of Rome, there weren't so many childless shepherds hanging about waiting for a chance to add to their family.

Not every exposed baby died; some probably found themselves in slavery and others maybe did find themselves picked up by a family in want of a child. Juvenal has a line that suggests that such a thing was possible, 'Spurious children, changelings picked up beside some filthy cistern and passed off as nobly born.'[3] But realistically a fair number would have starved to death.

There were numerous reasons why a child might be exposed, the most basic of which was as a form of family planning in an age where contraception was unreliable. Sick babies were certainly exposed, and the Greek doctor Soranus has a long list of what you should look for in a baby to ascertain whether it is worth rearing. He advises midwives to look for a vigorous crying infant. She should then check that the child's joints move as expected, that every part of its body looks how it should look and that there are no obstructions to any orifice. Emphasis is also placed on the health of a new-born being related to the mother's experience of pregnancy and her health, as well as being born no earlier than nine months. Soranus closes his chapter with the brutal line, 'Conditions contrary to those mentioned, the infant not worth rearing is recognised.'[4]

Of those babies that were exposed, the greater number were female. As in other parts of the world even today, girls were considered more a burden than boys, unable to partake in the same type of money-making work and in need of a dowry when they were married. As dream interpreter Artemidorus neatly summarises, 'Once brought up the males are no cost to their parents, but the females require a dowry.'[5] It is significant that to dream of a having a daughter signified financial loss and debt, whereas to dream of a male baby signified a good outcome.

A letter from Egypt, dated to the first century BCE, lays this chilling thinking bare. An absent husband, Hilarion, writes to his pregnant wife, Alis, 'If you have the baby before I return, if it is a boy let it live; if it is a girl; expose it.'[6]

Marriage was another institution where the paterfamilias had absolute power. The minimum age for marriage was twelve and most women would find themselves first married between the ages of twelve and fifteen. They had very little choice in who they married; this was determined by the paterfamilias, who could also dissolve her marriage if he so chose.[7]

The marriage market

Marriages and betrothals were, notably in the Late Republican era, made for political reasons. Given how tumultuous this period was politics wise, it's not surprising that these betrothals and marriages were in a similar state of flux.

A good example of this is Octavian, whose ever-changing betrothals matched the ever-changing political situation he found himself in after the assassination of his great uncle and adopted father, Julius Caesar. He was initially betrothed to Servilia, the daughter of the suitably impressive ex-consul, Publius Servilius Vatia Isauricus. However, needing to build an alliance with the most powerful man in Rome at the time, Mark Antony, Octavian broke off this betrothal to form a betrothal with Antony's stepdaughter, Claudia.

This second betrothal, however, became less attractive after Claudia's mother, Fulvia, went to war against him and so Octavian broke it off and betrothed himself instead to Scribonia. She happened to be a relative of Sextus Pompey, a troublesome pirate who was causing him no end of trouble at the time. This betrothal actually led to a marriage, a very unhappy marriage which Octavian gladly dissolved on the very day Scribonia gave birth to his daughter, Julia.

The timing may make us wince, but there was a reason why Octavian was so keen to ditch Scribonia; he wanted to marry Livia Drusilla. At face value there appears little political capital in marrying Livia, not least because she was married and pregnant at the time (which caused considerable scandal). Her family, far from being useful allies, had sided with Julius Caesar's assassins. However, Livia's family, the Claudians, had been both influential and instrumental in Rome's history going back centuries. Octavian, on the other hand, could claim kinship to Julius Caesar through his inferior maternal line, though he has precious few impressive family members on his paternal line. His father had been the first in the family to be admitted to the Senate. As Antony taunted, Octavian was 'the grandson of a rope maker'.

On the surface, this unlikely marriage to Livia may well have been less about love and more a canny political move from one of history's canniest political movers. It also proved to be a long marriage, over fifty years, fitting neatly into Octavian's later guise as Augustus the holder of Rome's traditional morals and promoter of marriage.

Similar political manoeuvring can be found in the marriage of Julia, Julius Caesar's daughter, to Pompey. Julia was thirty years younger than her new husband, but she bound the two most powerful men in Rome together. It was her untimely death in childbirth that was said to have led to a breakdown in relations between the two men, and ultimately a civil war.

Women were a useful political tool, their worth calculated by their family connections, though they had no say in these negotiations. The first century CE doctor Soranus rather neatly sums this up, 'Women are usually married for the sake of children and succession, and not for mere enjoyment.'[8]

Whereas men could throw off the restrictions of their paterfamilias when he died, women were subject to control for the rest of their lives. On the death of their father a guardian would be appointed. This guardian oversaw her financial affairs and had to be present for such actions as buying or selling land, accepting an inheritance, making a will and other important transactions.

The role of guardian could be ripe for abuse or exploitation or just straightforward theft, which is why there were laws in place to protect women from guardians with nefarious motives, 'A man who contracts matrimony with his own female ward in violation of the Decree of the Senate is not legally married.'[9]

That women found this irritating is illustrated by one of the carrots of the Augustan morality legislation – pop out three children and you could ditch the male guardian.

What women should be – examples to live and die from

Alongside legal restrictions, there was a keen notion of what a woman should be and what qualities she should exhibit. A good indicator of what a 'good' woman was to Roman eyes can be found in epithets – which, naturally, are only going to stress the positive attributes of the deceased – such as this example: 'She who proceeded me in my death was my one and only wife, chaste in body, with a loving spirit, she lived faithful to her faithful husband, always optimistic, even in bitter times she never shirked her duty.'[10] Or 'I alive was called Aurelia Philematio, chaste, modest, ignorant of the foul ways of the crowd, faithful to my husband.'

Notice the word 'chaste': the chastity of women was peculiarly important to both the Roman male and the Roman state, as is shown in the tales of heroines from the Republican era. One such woman was Lucretia whose loss of chastity was the catalyst for the fall the monarchy that had ruled Rome since its founding by Romulus.

Sacrificing for virtue: Lucretia

In the sixth century BCE Rome was ruled by kings. The seventh of these kings was the aptly named Tarquin Superbus. Superbus meant arrogant and Tarquin was certainly that. Cruel and despotic, he was far from popular, but it took Lucretia to finally stir the people into a full-scale revolt against him.

One drunken night, the king's son, Sextus, got into a heated debate with friends over whose wife was the most perfect. His drinking buddy, Collatinus, was full of praise for his wife, Lucretia, declaring that no other woman could surpass her for both virtue and beauty. There was only one way to settle this argument, so off they rode into the night to check out how excelling Lucretia truly was.

They found her quietly weaving wool in the lamplight. She was indeed beautiful, and it was at this moment that Sextus formed a wicked lust for his friend's wife, alongside a determination to taint her evident virtue. A few days later, unbeknownst to Collatinus, he returned to the house, slipped into her bed chamber and, holding a sword to her throat, raped Lucretia.

When Sextus had departed, Lucretia called for her husband. He arrived with his friend, Lucius Junius Brutus. Lucretia with tears in her eyes explained what had happened. She made the two men pledge that Sextus would be punished, and as the men consoled her, she replied, 'I do not absolve myself from punishment; not in time to come shall ever unchaste woman live through the example of Lucretia.[11]

Taking a knife she had hidden in her clothing, she then stabbed herself in her breast. Brutus then makes a very inspiring speech about freedom and liberty and the evil of kings. It is very stirring, look it up. But we are not concerned with Brutus, let us return to Lucretia, for alongside Brutus the Liberator (a nickname he acquires for his king-quashing efforts) she is hailed as an example to live by (or more accurately die by). As she says herself above, she will not set the example for other women that you may carry on as normal after losing your chastity, even if it was taken by force.

Why Lucretia yields to Sextus' rape attempt, according to Livy, is just as interesting. It is not the threat of death that Sextus initially makes, as she is quite prepared to die rather than submit to him. But rather it is his threat that he will murder his own slave and lay the corpse beside her own body, so it would appear that she had committed adultery with the lowest of the low.

This adherence to her honour and her position in society, alongside her unwillingness to live with anything less than complete and utter faithful chastity, is what elevates Lucretia to the status of a heroine. Here we see the female equivalent of that slippery word, *virtus*, but here uniquely tied to sexual behaviour.

Appearance is greater than deeds: Verginia

A somewhat similar story to that of Lucretia appears elsewhere in Livy's History of Rome. This story is set in the fifth century BCE, so still within a period of their history that the Romans saw as predating their corruption by outside influences, wealth and immorality.

Verginia was the daughter of a respected plebeian family recently betrothed to a heroic tribune. Beautiful and in the bloom of her youth she took the fancy of a certain Appius Claudius. He set out to win her with those tried and tested instruments of seduction, presents and promises. However, Verginia, being a girl of high virtue, could not be corrupted and she rejected Appius Claudius' advances.

There now follows a legal saga worthy of a Sunday night TV drama. Knowing that Verginia's father was away with the army, Appius induced a friend of his to claim that she, Verginia, was his slave and had been born in his household, stolen and transferred to the house of Verginius. Verginia and her maids were escorted from the Forum by an associate of the decemvir [12] to court where Appius' pal told his absurd tale in front of a judge. The judge's verdict was that the girl's father should be summoned to answer these charges, but, until he arrived Verginia should stay with Appius' friend who claimed she was his slave.

Understandably, this did not go down well with Verginia's fiancée who made an impassioned speech, the gist of which was that he would do for Appius if anything happened to his betrothed. Again, what is interesting is the stress on chastity and honour: 'I am going to marry this maiden, and I am determined to have a chaste wife,'[13] says the fiancée. Yes, he's prepared to defend her until her father arrives, but he's very much thinking of his situation, 'I will vindicate her liberty at the price of my life, sooner than sacrifice my honour.'[14]

The mood between the two camps was getting heated and, sensing an imminent mob, Appius Claudius' relented and allowed Verginia to be taken into the care of her relatives until her father arrived. Verginius arrived the next day and all decamped back to the court where the arguments were put before the judge. To the shock of all, the judge's verdict was that Verginia, as Appius claimed, was a slave and not the daughter of Verginius.

Dumbfounded, Verginius begged that he speak with his daughter. The judge agreed and Verginius went with the girl, now deemed a slave, to a quiet area to speak. Once there he pulled out a butcher's knife and stabbed her in the breast. His defence? As Verginia could no longer live in chastity he felt it preferable that she should die rather than be dishonoured. As in the case of Lucretia, death here is preferable to the shame of being unchaste and a woman's chastity, in both cases, has a major impact on the state. In Lucretia's case it brought down a monarchy, in Verginia's it led to the abolition of the decemvirs after Verginius marched his men on the city and demanded justice.

Let the Goddess prove my virtue: Claudia Quinta

Another tale of a woman's chastity being entwined with the state, and one that just about fits into our golden era, is that of Claudia Quinta.

During the time of the second Punic war,[15] Rome's fortunes suffered, most notably when the Roman forces were almost entirely wiped out by Hannibal's army at the Battle of Cannae.[16]

As a response to the terrible situation Rome found herself in, dreadful portents and omens were popping out of every crevice and a famine had stuck. Clearly the gods were not very happy. The Sibylline Oracle was consulted[17] and suggested that Rome's fortunes could be turned around if the goddess Cybele was added to the pantheon of gods. Cybele, also known as Magna Mater meaning 'Great Mother', was a cult that flourished in the east and hailed originally from Phrygia, in modern day Turkey. That the Romans were prepared to introduce a foreign goddess into their pantheon of gods show how truly desperate the situation was.

This new goddess was met at Ostia by a representative of the Roman state and a group of Roman matrons, including Claudia Quinta. These women were to tow the goddess to Rome. Claudia, though a chaste woman, was the subject of nasty gossips who claimed that chastity was a lie based on her clothes, her hairstyle and some unspecified behaviour.

Along her journey down the river Tiber, the goddess at one point got stuck in the mud. It was here that Claudia Quinta stepped forward, knelt down, undid that supposedly unchaste hairdo and beseeched the goddess, 'Kind and fruitful Mother of the Gods, accept a suppliant's prayers, on this one condition: They deny I'm chaste: let me be guilty if you condemn me: convicted by a goddess I'll pay for it with my life. But if I'm free of guilt, grant a pledge of my innocence by your action: and, chaste, give way to my chaste hands.'[18] She then picked up the tow rope and pulled. Miraculously the goddess became instantly unstuck in the mud and drifted along behind Claudia all the way to her new home in Rome.

This tale has the same hallmarks as that of Lucretia and Verginia: Claudia, if she is proven to be unchaste, will forfeit her life. But it more explicitly links a woman's sexual behaviour with the state and state religion. Claudia's chastity pleases the goddess, so she complies.

The health of the state was dependent on the happiness of the gods, if the gods were not happy then they must be appeased, or a reason found for this unhappiness. Sometimes that unhappiness was laid directly at the feet of women, none more so than in the case of the Vestal Virgins.

Keeping the fire burning: Vestal Virgins

The Vestals were priestesses charged with keeping the sacred flame of Vesta burning. They served in post for thirty years during which they enjoyed more rights than other Roman women, including a front seat at the games[19] and freedom from a male guardian. They took an oath of chastity upon taking up the position and so important was their chastity that there was a particularly horrible punishment awaiting any Vestal who broke it: being buried alive.

Although Roman law is scattered with horrible punishments it can be difficult sometimes to find any examples of such punishments being enacted. For example, in the Twelve Tables of Roman law that date back to the early Republican era, it is stated that a debtor can be physically torn apart by their creditors, though there are no examples to be found of this happening. Without a police force in place deterrents for crime needed to be seen to be harsh, hence their extreme nature. But we do know that some Vestals were executed in exactly this manner.

Executed is perhaps the wrong word; it is more of a trial, not unlike the one Claudia Quinta faced. A chaste Vestal would surely be saved by the goddess, an unchaste one would die entombed. Roman history has it that at least one Vestal disproved the charge levied against her by way of divine intervention and her name was Tuccia.

Like Claudia Quinta, Tuccia prayed to a goddess to prove her chastity. She would be proved pure if she could draw water from the river Tiber with a sieve and carry it without spillage to the Temple of Vesta. Events turned sensational when Tuccia carried her full sieve of water to the Forum without a drop being spilled. The goddess Vesta had proved Tuccia innocent of all charges.

There is another accusation of chastity breaking thrown at the Vestals in this era, one that does not have a happy ending. This one took place during Rome's lowest point in the second Punic war, the same period that Cybele was brought to Rome. The city was beset with terrible prodigies and Livy lists amongst these portents the broken chastity of two Vestals, Opimia and Floronia. Opimia had been buried alive, Floronia had committed suicide. This, alongside other disasters, was considered so dire that Quintus Fabius Pictor was despatched to Delphi to consult the famous oracle to ask what prayers and offerings the gods needed to restore Rome's fortunes.

It appears from this tale, and that of Tuccia, that during times when Rome faced great peril the chastity of the Vestals came under suspicion as a direct cause of upsetting the city's protecting gods.

The Vestals might also find themselves targeted by an emperor keen to take a moral stance. This is certainly what Pliny the Younger felt about an event he witnessed under the reign of Domitian, 'That emperor had determined that Cornelia, chief of the Vestal Virgins, should be buried alive, from an extravagant notion that exemplary severities of this kind conferred lustre upon his reign.'[20]

As in the case of Tuccia and Claudia Quinta, Cornelia cried out to the gods for help in proving her innocence, declaring that she couldn't possibly be guilty given the success of the emperor's reign. She had a point. In the late first century CE Rome was settled, peaceful and prosperous: certainly not a city in dire peril as in previous centuries.

Pliny is unable to say for definite whether Cornelia was innocent or guilty of the charge. But he does say from what he personally witnessed that she preserved the appearance of innocence, particularly in the final moments before her entombment. As she was being lowered down to her death her dress caught on something, and the executioner began to help free it, but she turned to him with a look of horror on her face, pulling herself away from being so much as touched by a man.

Cornelia may well have been the innocent victim of politics, and this ran true for those on the other side of the accusation as well. There are several instances in our sources of high-ranking men being accused and charged with breaking the chastity of a Vestal, with one example being the richest man in Rome during the Late Republican era, Marcus Licinius Crassus. The convicted lover of a Vestal could expect a public scourging. This involved a thorough and bloody beating with rods to the death, and in the case of Cornelia's alleged lovers, this took place in the Forum.

Even if it did not go to trial and a conviction, being accused of dalliances with a Vestal was drawing attention to a defect in your character. We are back with the Romans' obsession over the private life reflecting the public man. Whereas for a Vestal to lose her chastity was to endanger the fabric of society itself, for the accused man it showed a reckless disregard for the sacristy of the gods, of putting his pleasure first before the state. How could such a man be trusted as a public official when he would so readily abandon the gods for a quick shag?

This is amply demonstrated by the Emperor Elagabalus, whose tally of depravities is barely believable. Just when you think he can't sink any lower it is thrown in that he violated the chastity of a Vestal and even married her. Firmly linked to this sexual transgression is one against the state: Elagbalus raided and stole from the temple of Vesta, as the Historia Augusta very strongly puts it, 'by removing the holy shrines he profaned the sacred rites of the Roman nation.'[21]

Alongside chastity there were other virtues that Romans felt women should possess, such as self-sacrifice. Pliny the Younger recounts the oddly disturbing tale of a wife whose husband was suffering greatly with what Pliny calls ulcers in the private parts. Begging her husband to show her the damage (considerable), the wife determined that she was soon to be a widow. Rather than sit by her husband's bed being a consoling presence at these very final moments of his life, she urges him to commit suicide. Clearly this verbal urging did not have the desired effect because, '[She] led him to his death herself, and forced him to follow her example by roping herself to him and jumping into the lake.'[22] An act that is not so much euthanasia but wholesale murder, yet Pliny admires this action greatly.

He also cites the example of Arria, whose fame seemed to be based on her repeated suicide attempts, complete with pithy one liner. Her first 'glorious deed' was to plunge a dagger into her breast after the death of her son, hand the bloody implement to her husband, saying, 'It does not hurt, Paetus.'[23] An excellent one liner, I'm sure you'll agree.

Later in Arria's life, Paetus is involved in a revolt. Both husband and wife are brought before the Emperor Claudius and it's looking grim for them. So Arria makes it even grimmer, and not waiting to see what her punishment will be (presumably, not that bad given she's of senatorial rank)[24] she leaps out of her chair and runs head first into the wall opposite, doing some nastiness to her skull, though not enough to stop her injecting another pithy line, 'I told you,' she said, 'that I should find a hard way to die if you denied me an easy one.'

If we set aside Arria's final actions, which were to do with her imminent likely execution, there is a recurring theme in these two tales from Pliny. Both Arria and the unnamed resident of Lake Como (who Pliny feels should be much better known) see death as preferable to living without a husband and a son. Which taps into what Roman men think is a woman's place in a society, as an appendage to men. Without those men, she may as well die for she is nothing on her own.

A less extreme example of a woman's value being firmly rooted in the requirements of men is found in a very touching inscription from the first century BCE. The *Laudatio Turiae* is a eulogy by a husband to his wife, Turia detailing their life together and all the times she was of assistance to him.

This being the time of the civil wars that wrecked Rome after the assassination of Julius Caesar, Turia's wifely deeds are a reflection of the difficult times they were both living in. For instance, we are told that the day before their wedding Turia's parents were both murdered, but being a dutiful daughter, she made sure their killers were punished. This is clearly not just a matter of reporting the issue to the local magistrate and watching the wheels of justice turn, since after the guilty verdict is passed Turia has to immediately vacate her home in order to 'protect her modesty,' which is altogether disturbing.

Even more disturbing is that Turia is later forced to beat back a gang of men intent on plundering their home.[25] Not to mention the time she begged for her husband's life by prostrating herself before Octavian's then colleague in power, Marcus Lepidus. She was dragged away 'like a slave,' says her husband, which we may interpret as a rough exit, one that had Turia covered in bruises. All in all, Turia spends her married life advising and protecting her husband, sometimes physically.

Turia and her husband have no children, and here her absolute dedication to the cause of her husband comes into play once again as she offers a solution for her barrenness. 'You proposed a divorce outright and offered to yield our house free to another woman's fertility.'

Turia's duty to her husband is such that she would give up her position as his wife and live subserviently to his new wife. To his credit, this unnamed husband is absolutely horrified by this suggestion, the marriage is not dissolved and Turia and her husband apparently live happily ever after.

The sister of Augustus, Octavia, displays a not dissimilar dedication to duty against her own interests after the death of her former husband, Antony, and his wife, Cleopatra. While her brother takes out (murders) Caesarian, Cleopatra's son by Julius Caesar, Octavia opts to raise Antony and Cleopatra's remaining children. This elevates her as a paragon of virtue.

What all these stories show is what the Romans admired in women was an excessive duty to the family. Whereas the Roman ideal male had an obligation to the public sphere, such as Cincinnatus throwing off his plough to go and do his duty, the Roman ideal woman was busy fulfilling duties in the private sphere of the home and family.

We have seen how the law and cultural attitudes shaped how Roman men thought women should behave, but did they?

Real women of Rome

The Lucretias of the world, much like Cincinnatus on the male side, were an ideal that few would ever achieve. Roman male writers looked back at women from the past, who may never have existed, and used them to attack the women of the present.

Finding examples of the behaviour of real-life women is harder than for men; they don't have handy biographies written about their achievements[26] and you don't tend to read about them in the lines of histories unless they do something extraordinarily dire. Instead we can piece together bits of their lives from other sources, such as inscriptions and dedications.

One hugely important and illustrative source we have is the staff list of Augustus' wife, Livia. Not only does it offer a valuable insight into the types of jobs that slaves in the imperial household held, it also demolishes a particular story put about by Augustus. Augustus, as we have seen previously, was keen on restoring traditional values and roles for women. We are told that, 'he wore common clothes for the house, made by his sister, wife, daughter or granddaughters.'[27]

The image he was projecting is your Cato the Elderesque humble living, resisting the temptation of luxury and maintaining a household in the traditional manner. Earlier in the chapter we saw Lucretia's wool spinning as part of what made her an excellent wife, the subtext being that if you are busy at home with your wool you're not getting into trouble in the dangerous city.

Livia's staff list, however, completely contradicts this propaganda. She employed (amongst many others it has to be said) a wool weigher, shoemaker, clothes mender, servant in charge of shrine clothes, servant in charge of purple clothes, servant in charge of ceremonial dress, a dresser, a servant in charge of whatever clothes were left and a clothes folder. This is not humble living. This is very far from humble living.

Satirist Juvenal dedicates his sixth satire to detailing absolutely everything he dislikes about the women of his era (the late first century CE). This turns out to be rather a lot. It is quite the rant and impossible to read without picturing Juvenal reciting it himself and getting ever redder in the face as the rage consumes him. But from this rather unpleasant misogyny we can piece together a picture of Roman women, most particularly those of the elite class, which paints a very different picture to those endlessly noble women who would rather die than dent their chastity.

The women of Juvenal's day were educated and well read. He is satisfyingly furious at women who at dinner parties quote poets he's never heard of and talk knowledgably about Virgil and Homer. He is enraged by women keeping up to date with current affairs, discussing the latest world news from Armenia, Thrace or Parthia. He finds it unbearable that women were often the instigators of court cases and took a keen interest in the legal proceedings, making suggestions to their lawyers.

The women in Juvenal attend the theatre, the circus, the amphitheatre, dinner parties and festivals, they go shopping and enjoy time at the baths, as well as carrying out copious affairs, according to Juvenal. These were certainly not Lucretias, at home weaving, waiting for the return of their husbands.

Elsewhere we find women owning and running businesses. From an urn we know of Sellia Epyre, who ran a successful enterprise manufacturing garments decorated with gold, a high-end business that was located on the exclusive Via Sacre which ran into the Forum.

The businesswoman: Eumachia

Pompeii has proved a rich treasure trove of information on the activities of women in the first century CE. Women's names are stamped onto bricks and pipes, showing them as the owner of the operation. Eumachia was one such woman.

She had become extremely wealthy from the family brick-making business, and just like the men of the time, she had used some of this money to finance public works. An enormous building in the Forum bears her name and an inscription telling us it was erected at her expense. At the far end there is even a statue of her that was funded and installed by the guild of fullers, of which she was patron. Eumachia also served as a priestess. Despite not being able to vote or stand for public office, Eumachia was nonetheless heavily involved in the public life of the town.

Other ways in which women were involved in public life in Pompeii can be seen in the electioneering graffiti which covered the walls of the city. There are over 2,000 such posters in Pompeii and several of them mention women's names or groups of women endorsing one candidate or another.

As well as patronage and throwing money about we do find some women in public roles and having influence at the highest level.

The eunuch dresser: Calvia Crispinilla

Calvia Crispinilla is a woman who gets a sneering reference in our written sources. She certainly does not resemble in any way the ideal of the elite Roman woman we've looked at so far. She took up the role of Nero's mistress of the wardrobe with the responsibility of dressing his favourite eunuch, Sporus. Linked with the excesses of the dying days of that reign, the historian Tacitus calls her Nero's 'tutor in vice'.[28]

After Nero was forced into suicide many former prominent members of his court were targeted for retribution. Calvia escaped this by journeying to Africa. Here she hooked up with a Roman official by the name of Clodius Macer, who does something rather surprising and sudden. He blockades the grain ships that sailed from Egypt to Rome and which fed the city. Tacitus is very clear that this revolt, for this is what it was, was entirely at the instigation of Calvia.

Presumably the idea of the blockade was to force Rome to bargain with Macer. Was he after money? Or perhaps he fancied himself as emperor. He does produce coinage with a picture of himself wearing a laurel wreath, which is highly suggestive. Ultimately, we don't know what Macer's endgame was since his plan, whatever it was, failed and he was executed by Nero's successor, Galba.

Calvia, however, despite being the instigator of a revolt against Galba and despite being one of Nero's closest aids,[29] escapes execution and all other forms of punishment. She does this by making a very advantageous marriage. We know not to whom, though Tacitus says a senior statesman but does not name him, suggesting he was still alive and influential in the historian's own time.

Calvia Crispinilla survives when so many of Nero's advisors did not and we are told that she retained the influence she held in those days through successive reigns. Tacitus intriguingly says this was down to her being a wealthy woman without heirs, adding 'for, whether times are good or bad, such qualities retain their power.'[30]

The restrictions placed upon women in ancient Rome would suggest that they have no role in public life, yet here we have Calvia Crispinilla, a woman of the senatorial class, working for an emperor, instigating a political coup, wriggling out of any repercussions and continuing to be powerful in her sphere. On top of this we know from the stamps on amphora recovered from a sunken ship that she was involved in the production of olive oil, probably through owning large estates.

We have seen that Roman women ran businesses, were educated, knowledgeable on literature and current affairs and served in some forms of public office – all contrary to that ideal we explored earlier in the chapter. Similarly, the Lucretia ideal of extreme chastity or death does not hold up terribly well either.

Juvenal, alongside his complaints about women being cleverer than him, has a long list of sexual violations too. Juvenal writes satire and so we should always keep in mind that his stories are exaggerated for comic effect, but for satire to work it must be based on a recognisable truth. And with that disclaimer, let us go back to the nineties CE and see what Juvenal's contemporaries were up to.

'During Saturn's reign I believe that Chastity still lingered on earth and was seen for a while,'[31] so Juvenal says, and then proceeds to demolish the morals of his own time. The women who spent time at the games and the theatre were not there for the culture or entertainment, according to Juvenal. No, they are all lusting after the actors and half-naked gladiators. Music lessons bring with them music teachers, and a quite different instrument to play with. A trip to the public baths brings the opportunity for a 'happy ending' courtesy of the talented hands of the masseur. Mothers-in-law enjoy their slaves, and widows take advantage of those legacy hunters swarming around them. Everyone is at it!

It's invective, it's rhetoric with a swagger, but to be funny these tales of women lusting after actors and having flings with slaves at least had to possess a crumb of plausibility. From which we might conclude that women had the means, motive and opportunity for sexual dalliances if they chose. They certainly weren't tied to the home weaving all day, as Roman men would have liked them to be.

Chapter 5

Neither Male nor Female

We have seen how the Romans had very strong opinions on what made a man and what made a woman. But there were people who fell between the cracks, being neither one nor the other. 'There are people who have the characteristics of both sexes. We call them hermaphrodites. Once considered portents, now they are sources of entertainment.'[1]

'Sources of entertainment' is a very Roman thing, they adored anything out of the ordinary, particularly when it was presented in human form. Pliny tells us about Gabbara of Arabia who stood at 10ft tall and toured the empire when Claudius was emperor. The Emperor Domitian always kept with him a small boy with an oversized head who was said to advise him on great matters. There were 'novelty' gladiator bouts set between the blind and disabled. Hermaphrodites fall into the same category.

Hermaphrodites

The original Hermaphrodite features in Greek myth; born male, he was the child of Hermes and Aphrodite. Given his great resemblance to both his parents, his name was an amalgamation of their names, Hermaphroditus.

Hermaphroditus' life was changed when the water nymph Salmacis fell in instant lust with him. She dragged him into her pond, merging their forms together to be both male and female at the same time.

Hermaphroditus is the subject of numerous pieces of art, most notably 'The Sleeping Hermaphroditus', which you will have seen a copy of if you have ever wandered around any great museum. The Louvre in Paris, the Borghese in Rome, the Hermitage in St Petersburg, the Metropolitan Museum in New York amongst others, all contain a version of this statue (see image 7).

The statue depicts Hermaphroditus lying on their side, from one angle you see the rounded buttocks and breast swell of a woman. Scoot round the other side, however, and your view is changed entirely as Hermaphroditus' male tackle is exposed resting on the couch. This surprise elicits smiles and laughs as your preconceptions are swept from under your feet.

That there are quite so many modern copies of 'The Sleeping Hermaphroditus' shows the lasting appeal of the unexpected. The humour likely worked the same way in ancient Rome, with the host enjoying his guests' reactions when the secret of his statue was revealed.

Sex changes

Hermaphroditus was not alone in altering his biological sex from that he was born with. Pliny the Elder has a whole chapter entitled 'Changes of Sex'. He begins this by saying, 'That women have changed into men is not a myth,'[2] and proceeds to give examples where this had happened.

Pliny tells us of a girl from Casinum, in northern Italy, who turned into a boy before her parents' 'very eyes'. He has found the evidence for this amazing transformation in the historical records and even has a date for when this sex change occurred, 171 BCE.

Licinius Mucianus is his source for the tale of Arescon, who had once been a woman named Arescusa. She had even been married, but after the wedding had slowly obtained the characteristics of a man, including a sizeable beard. We must assume that her husband was less than pleased with this, because when Mucianus met Arescon/Arescusa he was now married to a woman. Pliny sees no reason to doubt Mucianus' story and we have no reason to either.

Mucianus was a wealthy, highly respected Roman politician with no need to sell apocryphal stories for cash. He was level-headed enough in 69 CE to realise he was not emperor material and instead helped the very practical Vespasian to the throne. While Vespasian made his way from the East to claim the purple, Mucianus ran Rome successfully in his absence. If Mucianus records he met a man who told him he had once been a woman, then I think we can deduce that is exactly what happened. Whether Arecusa/Arescon is quite so reliable is another question entirely.

However, these corroborated tales of sex changes pale into insignificance alongside this: 'In Africa, I myself saw someone who became a man on his wedding day.'[3] Yes, Pliny himself witnessed first-hand someone change sex, with the added drama that this took place on their wedding day. Now here is our evidence, our fully documented account, except that it's not because this is, unforgivably, the only details Pliny gives us. It should be noted that he dedicates no fewer than eighteen chapters to bees and honey. But about the wedding he attended where the bride became a man, one solitary line.

From a medical/biological view, obviously all these stories are impossible, women cannot physically turn into men spontaneously, but that is not the point. The point is that the Romans believed they were possible. This tells you something of how they understood the differences between men and women, that they were not as concrete, as immovable as you might have thought from the clearly defined gender roles we looked at in the last two chapters.

Eunuchs

Hermaphroditus was intersex through his bodily merging with the water nymph. We have looked at those who were said to have spontaneously changed sex, but there were another group of people who fell between the sexes, being neither male nor female: eunuchs.

There were evidently two methods of castration available in the ancient world. The first involved an incision made in the scrotum and the testes removed. The second involved the would-be eunuch being sat in a bath of hot water and the testes squeezed until they disappear. The second method by compression was only possible on children where the testicles had not fully developed.[4] These types of eunuchs are sometimes referred to in sources as *thlibias*, meaning 'to press', or *thladias* meaning 'to crush'.

We find mention of eunuchs scattered across Roman society, including within the imperial household. The Emperor Claudius gets a bashing in the sources for his promotion of the eunuch Posides, who was evidently given some great honour at Claudius' British triumph. Juvenal scorns at his home which apparently outshone the emperor's own.

Another eunuch, Halotos, served as Claudius' food taster. A job he singularly failed at, given Claudius died after being poisoned. Or perhaps he had another master, for he certainly prospered during the reign of Claudius' successor, Nero.

Evidently the number of imperial eunuchs underwent a certain amount of inflation because during the reign of the Emperor Alexander Severus, 222–235 CE, we find policies being enacted to restrict their numbers. 'Whereas Elagabalus had been the slave of his eunuchs, Alexander reduced them to a limited number and removed them from all duties in the Palace except the care of the women's baths; and whereas Elagabalus had also placed many over the administration of the finances and in procuratorships, Alexander took away from them even their previous positions.'[5]

This clearly does nothing to restrict the ever-increasing influence of eunuchs at court, and by the reign of Constantine the Great's son, Constanius II, in the fourth century, they are highly influential. Most particularly the grand chamberlain, Eusebius, who Ammianus Marcellinus delightfully describes as being 'sufficiently inclined to mischief'.[6] In the fourth and fifth centuries we find eunuchs with a similar prominence to Eusebius operating with considerable influence over the emperors they supposedly served.

Eunuchs reach their zenith of authority and visibility in the Byzantine period, from the sixth century onwards. This is the era where we find eunuchs wielding great power in the position of grand chamberlain. This role, exclusively held by eunuchs, is on a par in rank with the praetorian prefect in charge of the emperor's bodyguards, which demonstrates quite how influential they could be.

Elsewhere we find eunuchs such as Theophilos leading military campaigns, stepping in for the emperor when he was away campaigning, as in the case of the eunuch Baanes, and being key in arranging the succession of the next emperor, as the eunuch Amantius was. This period is awash with stories of despicable, untrustworthy eunuchs double crossing and plotting at the highest levels. They were ubiquitous members of the imperial court.

Why were eunuchs particularly promoted to high ranking positions at court? Being an emperor is a dangerous job: you have an extremely high chance of being murdered, therefore it is important that you have staff around you whom you can trust. Because they lacked family, eunuchs were thought to possess greater loyalty to the emperor and the imperial family. A loyalty that was compounded by the dislike and distaste they attracted in the wider community, which isolated them from the rest of society. That was the theory; however, the history of eunuchs at court would appear to disprove this entirely as they were as ambitious and self-seeking as any other Roman male.

Aside from the superior position of grand chamberlain and similar roles, the enforced boyhood of eunuchs perhaps unsurprisingly made them sexual objects. That eunuchs were used for sex is clear from a second-century law which forbade the castration of men for purposes of debauchery and is amply proved by the praetorian prefect, Sejanus, who named his (ludicrously pricey)[7] eunuch Paezon, meaning boy toy, which is about as blatant as you can get. Although there is one other example that blows Paezon out of the water, Nero's favourite eunuch, Sporus.

The eunuch who would be empress: Sporus

The tale of Sporus is often used as the ultimate example of Nero's deranged depravity. In 65 CE, during an argument about staying late at the chariot races, Nero kicked his wife, Poppaea Sabina, in the stomach. Unfortunately, Poppaea was heavily pregnant at the time and the kick, despatched in a moment of anger, led to her death.

Nero was devastated by Poppaea's death, staging a magnificent state funeral for her during which more perfume was burned than Arabia produced in an entire year. Her body was embalmed with spices and Nero gave the oration himself on his deceased wife's many attributes.

His grief was such that on hearing there was a woman that greatly resembled Poppaea he sent for her. Evidently, she didn't resemble Poppaea enough since Nero soon tired of her and moved onto another clone of his wife, who this time was a boy.

We are told that Nero had the boy castrated and treated him in every way like Poppaea. He dressed this Poppaea clone in the finery of an empress and travelled with him in a litter through the streets of Rome. Nero addressed Sporus as 'Sabina', or empress. This empress accompanied Nero on his tour of Greece. In Delphi they went through a wedding ceremony complete with dowry and bridal veil, with the praetorian prefect Tigellinus giving the 'bride' away. Thrilled at hosting an imperial wedding on their shores, the Greeks threw a magnificent celebration for the newly married couple.

Of course, Nero was already married to wife number three, Statilia Messalina, who may well have been accompanying her husband on his Greek tour. Quite what she thought about her husband having a public marriage ceremony with his favourite eunuch is not recorded. More's the pity.

What was Nero up to? Was he so lost in grief at causing his wife's death that he genuinely believed Sporus was Poppaea? After all, the entire Greek trip was one long fantasy with the emperor winning 1,500 prizes in the Panhellenic Games, including the chariot race at the Olympic Games despite crashing his chariot and failing to finish. Was this wedding, this wife another such reality created and maintained by the palace staff?

There is perhaps a clue in Sporus' name, which translates as spunk or seed. How cruelly apt a name for a eunuch that didn't possess any. Which begs the question, was it a joke? Was castrating a boy, dressing him up as your dead wife and parading him round the city Nero's idea of fun?

There's a certain theatrical element here that is very Nero; the dressing up, the extravagant public kisses, the wedding. Also, this wasn't Nero's first 'unofficial' wedding. There had been a previous wedding and marriage, this time with his freedman Pythagorus. Only at that wedding Nero had been the bride not the groom, with Suetonius adding in the detail that the emperor imitated the cries of a maiden being deflowered on his wedding night.

This puts the Sporus wedding in another light. Was it a bit of play acting, a bit of sexual role play? Ultimately, we will never know. One thing is for sure though, Sporus was important to Nero. He was one of only three people Nero took with him during his final flight from Rome. The eunuch/wife was with his emperor when Nero stabbed himself with a dagger after he'd begged the eunuch to help him commit suicide by setting an example of how it should be done first. Sporus declined the offer to kill himself and Nero went to his death alone.

Sporus has a curious post-Nero life that muddies the story even further. After Nero's death he pops up in the company of Nymphidius Sabinus, the praetorian prefect who encouraged the guards to abandon the emperor. Sabinus, we are told, sent for Sporus while Nero's body was still burning on its pyre.

Previously we have considered that perhaps Nero was so grief-stricken he truly believed Sporus was Poppaea. If he did, it was a delusion that was spreading. Nymphidius Sabinus too referred to Sporus as Sabina, and, we are told, treated him as his consort, his empress. Surely Sabinus couldn't be sharing the same delusion as Nero?

Sabinus' actions do hint at a troubled mind. Left in charge of Rome while the new emperor, Galba, was in the provinces, he begins to get delusions of grandeur acting as if he were the emperor. When Galba got wind of Sabinus' antics and reprimanded him, the prefect took a truly astonishing route, he decided to declare himself emperor. He justified this new coup by claiming to be the son of Caligula and so possessed of a better claim to the title than Galba.

This was the thinking of a desperate or troubled man, possibly both, for even if this were true (and it's not entirely unfeasible given Sabinus' mother, Nymphidia, was a palace prostitute who was intimate with Caligula) he was illegitimate. Secondly, being the son of a previous emperor gave him no road to power as sons did not automatically inherit the imperial title. It wasn't until 79 CE that a father first handed power over to a son in Rome, when Titus succeeded Vespasian as emperor, and it didn't happen again until 180 CE with Commodus succeeding Marcus Aurelius.

Sabinus' own men saw the foolishness of his plan, even if he didn't. They stepped in to stop this coup by the tried and tested Roman method of dealing with politicians who go that bit too far, they hacked him to death.

But what of Sporus, what happened to him? Well, he pops up yet again playing the role of empress, this time to Otho. Otho proved far better at organising a coup than Sabinus and had overthrown Galba during one very bloody day of killing in January 69 CE. Again, Otho, like Nero and Sabinus before him, was said to have called Sporus Sabina, which has an added dimension of peculiarity here because Otho had been married to the actual Poppaea Sabina.

Otho's marriage to Poppaea had ended when Nero had taken a fancy to her and insisted his friend divorce his wife. Or alternatively, Otho had married Poppaea to provide a smokescreen of respectability while she and the emperor continued their affair, but then had unexpectedly fallen in love with her. In both scenarios Otho refuses to divorce Poppaea and is sent into exile. Well, sort of: he was made governor of Lusitania – modern-day Portugal –which some saw as the means of getting the jealous husband out the way and others saw as a reward from Nero for handing over his wife. There was even speculation that this had been a ménage à trois until Otho's feelings had unsettled the balance.

Things are no less confusing when Otho becomes emperor, because while consorting with Sporus and calling him by the name of his dead wife, Otho was also pursuing a relationship with Nero's widow, Statilia Messalina, and had plans to marry her. However, after only three months of rule, Otho's forces were defeated by the army of Vitellius and he committed suicide.

The now Emperor Vitellius sent for Sporus too, but his reasons for doing so were grim. He did not want Sporus as an empress or a consort, or even as a sparkly member of his court. Fond of the Games, Vitellius hit upon the idea of Sporus playing a key role in a staged reenactment of the rape of Proserpina. Sporus was having none of it and committed suicide rather than face the shame of such a public appearance.

Sporus' story, as we have seen, is a very odd one. There is not another eunuch who features quite so heavily in the historical narrative, until we get to the fourth century when eunuchs play a political role in the administration. It is difficult to know what to make of Sporus and his role. Was he the cruelly abused toy of a crazed emperor, brutally mutilated and forced to perform as a woman?

His presence with Nero at his end suggests he was more than a joke to that emperor. That Sabinus picks up where Nero left off suggests that Sporus played a blinder in the role of empress and had played it often enough for him to be a feasible consort. That Otho, who was extremely familiar with the original Poppaea, takes up with Sporus suggests his impersonation of the dead empress was extraordinarily good. The fact that Sporus commits suicide rather than perform for Vitellius strongly suggests that the eunuch did not see himself as an imperial servant to take orders or play a role. He was better than that.

There are a lot of ifs and maybes with the tale of Sporus, but I believe there is one thing we can say for certain, he must have made an extraordinarily attractive and convincing woman.

Oh sweetest boy: Earinus

Some twenty years after Sporus' sad demise the Emperor Domitian, enactor of a very many morality laws, is much taken by the eunuch Earinus.

Earinus, unlike Sporus, plays little part in the historical record but he is the subject of some very cloying verses from court poets Statius and Martial. Earinus is described by Statius as 'a bright star of unmatched beauty.' Martial says he is 'dearest to the emperor of all that compose his court.'

Both write poems about Earinus' coming of age when his hair was cut. Statius' poem begins, 'Go, locks of hair, go swiftly over favourable seas,' and it is downhill from there. Though you have to admire the sheer genius of Statius for integrating a poem on a court favourite with the emperor's recent anti-castration legislation.

> Had you been born later, you too, of greater strength,
> Would have known darkened cheeks, and fuller limbs.
> You'd have rejoiced to send beard as well as shavings
> To Apollo's shrine.[8]

Martial and Statius both compare Earinus and Domitian to the mythological couple Ganymede and Jupiter.

Ganymede was an attractive young boy who Jupiter kidnapped in the guise of an eagle and set him to work as his cup bearer in the heavens. The relationship between Jupiter and Ganymede is portrayed as a sexual one, notably in this line from the Aeneid, 'Jove's smile that beamed on eagle-ravished Ganymede.'[9] Which begs the question, was the relationship between Domitian and Earinus sexual too?

Earinus is certainly the recipient of some very flowery compliments on his appearance, but it doesn't necessarily follow that there was sex involved. Domitian was much attached to the god Jupiter, who he credited with saving his life during the civil war of 69 CE. Comparisons of Domitian to Jupiter are everywhere in the court poetry of the time; the Ganymede/Jupiter comparison could just be an extension of this.

In addition, it seems good form to describe all of Domitian's staff as attractive and brilliant, and this is the subject of several poems. Partly because their brilliance reflects on the brilliance of the emperor for employing them, but also because poets depended on the imperial freedman's influence to get their poems in front of the emperor.[10]

From Statius' poem and from Domitian's own legislation on castration we might deduce his interest in Earinus was one of pity for his state, though Suetonius claims that Domitian's laws were introduced purely to spite his brother, Titus, because of his well-known fondness for eunuchs. It's one hell of a pointless revenge given Titus was long dead.

That Earinus is not used as a means of knocking an unpopular emperor (which Domitian was in spades) is another indicator that this was not a sexual relationship. Although we should be clear that any 'relationship' was very one-sided: an emperor got what he wanted, his chosen partner had no choice.

Roman men were not the only ones who were drawn to the figure of the eunuch, there was also a suspicion that women were getting in on the action too. Juvenal is convinced the mincing gait of the eunuch is a disguise to hide his rampant virility. He suggests that eunuchs are a preferable lover as they have beardless chins for softer kisses and there is zero chance of getting pregnant by them. The eunuchs here are sex objects for the bored, horny housewife.

The priests of Cybele

Outside of imperial circles we find eunuchs involved in religion, most notably in the cult of the Great Mother, Cybele, and her consort, Attis. As with all myths, there are several versions of Attis' story, the one thing they all agree on is that he was an attractive boy from Phrygia; representations of Attis portray him wearing a Phrygian cap.[11] In one version the nymph Agdistis falls in love with Attis, but unfortunately for Agdistis, Attis was due to marry another. It is fair to say that Agdistis did not take this well and took the radical step of sending the wedding party insane, an insanity which led to Attis castrating himself with a piece of flint.

> "Ah! Let the parts that harmed me, perish!
> Let them perish!" cutting away the burden of his groin,
> And suddenly bereft of every mark of manhood.
> His madness set a precedent, and his unmanly servants
> Toss their hair, and cut off their members as if worthless.[12]

Another version has Attis' crazed self-mutilation caused by Cybele herself as punishment for his lapse in chastity with the nymph.

As a link to Attis' sad tale, the priests of Cybele, the Galli priests, were all eunuchs. This posed a problem for the Romans whose relationship with eunuchs can be summarised thus: they were nice things to have but not to be. It was unthinkable for any Roman male citizen of whatever class to submit to the knife, or even serve in any capacity such a clearly foreign cult. This conundrum was solved by importing Galli priests from the East.

The ban on Roman citizens serving in the Magna Mater cult was not the only restriction on the worship of Cybele. The Romans, fearful that this Eastern cult would infect Roman morals, effectively sealed the Galli off from interacting with society, and instead they stayed in their temple on the Palatine Hill until they were required. That requirement occurred each April with the Megalesia Festival.

Commencing on 4 April, the Megalesia was a six-day extravaganza of festival delights. The Galli priests let loose from their temple danced through the streets accompanied by tambourines and flutes, dressed in their saffron robes. They pulled an effigy of the goddess down to the Circus Maximus, after which the chariot races in her honour would begin.

The Galli's frenzied dancing and howling in imitation of Attis' madness must have been a strange sight for the population. On 10 April the goddess and her eunuchs would return to their sanctuary on the Palatine Hill and not be seen again until the following year.

The law

Although, as we have seen, there were eunuchs present in Rome throughout her history and there was some kudos in owning one, the Romans never got over their distaste for the castrated state. It was all a bit Eastern and decadent and it did not feel like it was something that they should be partaking in. This is why there were repeated attempts to legislate on the creation and status of eunuchs.

Domitian's morality laws in the late first century CE forbade the castration of any boy, freeborn or not freeborn, and then, knowing any limitation in availability would greatly please the bank balance of the slave dealers, he froze the amount of money that you could charge for a eunuch.

Evidently Domitian's laws either did not last or were not having the proposed effect because we find the Emperor Hadrian introducing a law forbidding entirely the castration of boys. What is interesting about Hadrian's law, intriguing even, is that there is a recognition that some people were a willing party in castration. 'No one has a right to castrate a freeman or a slave, either against his consent or with it, and no one can voluntarily offer himself to be castrated. If anyone should violate my Edict, the physician who performed the operation shall be punished with death, as well as anyone who willingly offered himself for emasculation.'[13] Which begs the question, who on earth was willingly offering themselves up for castration and why? Were they frenzied followers of Attis and Cybele wishing to enter the Galli? Was there money to be made in being castrated? It is infuriatingly mysterious.

Punishments for playing any part in a castration are straightforward and harsh: death for most involved. Clearly they had little effect on stopping the practise because in the third century CE those legal minds are puzzling out questions relating to a eunuch's status: 'Eunuchs can make a will at the time when most males arrive at the age of puberty, that is to say, when they have reached their eighteenth year.'[14] Evidently there was a market for eunuchs that defied all imperial attempts to crush it.

Chapter 6

How to be Sexy: Beauty and Fashion

Having examined in our previous chapters the characteristics that made an ideal citizen of Rome, we shall now get distinctly more superficial by concentrating on the exterior. What was considered beautiful in ancient Rome? What did a Roman man or woman look for in a partner? And how might you go about upping your gorgeousness level in the hope of captivating and indeed capturing a lover?

Enhancing beauty

'You need to be attractive when men these days are so debonair, Your husbands dress up to the nines like ladies, a bride has hardly smarter things to wear.'[1]

The ideal Roman man was one devoid of vanity in his appearance, a rugged fellow busy working the land only pausing to undertake crucially important work for the state. The ideal Roman woman had no need of vanity either, she was happily married and far too busy spinning wool to think of her looks.

However, in the real world, outside of the imagined golden age, both men and women put an awful lot of time, money and thought into their appearance. We know this because it is the subject of endless scorn from the likes of Juvenal, but let us put the moaning to one side for the time being and look at what an ancient Roman beauty routine consisted of.

The poet Ovid is the surprising author of work entitled 'Cosmetics for Women', which demonstrates the effort Roman women were expected to put into their appearance,

> Beauty's a gift of the gods: how many can boast it?
> The larger number among you lack such gifts.
> Taking pains brings beauty: beauty neglected dies.[2]

Ovid's cosmetics certainly involve taking pains: his recommended face cream, for example, consists of barley, ten eggs, ground stag antler, twelve narcissus bulbs, two ounces of Tuscan seed and honey. The fact that instructions are also given on how to prepare it (including the measured quantities) shows that Ovid expected this face cream to be homemade.

No lower-class woman of Rome had the time to collect such an exhausting list of ingredients, nor wrestle a stag and saw off its antlers, let alone pound them into dust. No, Ovid's make-up tips were aimed very much at the elite woman, and her slaves, for they would be the ones peeling narcissus bulbs one after the other.

That this is aimed solely at upper-class women is shown by Ovid's descriptions of the women he knows; they have gowns with hems of gold and are adorned with jewels. Certainly not the wife of your local butcher.

Ovid's labour-intensive beauty products concentrate, in the main, on complexion. Freckles are deemed to be bad and must be covered up with a paste made from a bird's nest mixed with honey. A lovely fresh complexion could be gained from a potion made from incense, peeled gum, myrrh, fennel, rose petals, frankincense and barley liquid; which must have been ruinously expensive.

After all that, though, it seems beauty comes from within, as Ovid declares, 'your first thought, ladies should be for your behaviour, a face will please when character is fine.' So much for that ground stag antler!

Elsewhere we find other suggestions on improving your complexion. To prevent wrinkles asses' milk was used, presumably this was rubbed into the skin. Although Nero's wife, Poppaea, took it one step further by bathing in it, presumably to show off her imperial status that meant she had slaves to spare for ass-milking duties. Another animal-related face product that pops up several times is crocodile dung. The mind (and presumably the nose) boggles!

A bread poultice was meant to soften the skin and the plant helenium was thought to not only produce a bright complexion but also to increase a woman's sex appeal, while curing asthma and banishing sorrow at the same time. Helenium is quite the wonder plant.[3]

A pale skin was the preferred complexion since it showed that you were wealthy and idle enough not to have to work outdoors. A popular way to achieve this look was by using *cerussa* (sugar of lead): vinegar was poured over white lead shavings, dissolving them, and the remnants were then dried, ground together and fashioned into a tablet. Alternatives were available to this face-rotting foundation, such as clay mixed with calcium carbonate known as *melinum* and chalk dust mixed with vinegar.

Evidently some women went too far with the make-up. Juvenal sneers at faces, 'Caked with layers of bread-paste, reeking of greasy Poppaean Creams, that stick to her wretched husband's lips.'[4]

Less lethal than white lead was the kohl or saffron that was applied round the eyes, green malachite which served as eye shadow and poppies or ochre, if you afford it, to colour lips and cheeks a luscious red.

The important thing for Ovid about all this beautifying is that it should be done in private. You must keep that bedroom door closed, and you must hide your bottles and powders because men should never know of this process. Perhaps this explains why our male writers are so singularly unappreciative of all the efforts their womenfolk have gone through on their behalf: they have no clue as to the time, expense and hard work involved.

Perfume

'Perfume is the most pointless of all luxuries, their highest recommendation is that, as a woman goes by their use may attract event those who are otherwise occupied.'[5]

As you might gather from the quote above, Pliny the Elder is not a fan of perfume, in fact, he is uncharacteristically furious about perfume. Who knew that perfume was so contentious a subject?

The reason that Pliny is so furious about perfume is that it is linked very much to the luxury that he, and many others, believed was responsible for the moral decline of Rome. Interestingly, Pliny's *Natural History* has a chapter with the title 'The decay of morality is caused by the produce of the sea', so we may at least absolve perfume from that.[6]

Perfume was fashionably expensive, so fashionably expensive that the elite enter a game of competitive showing off. It was not enough for women to dab a bit behind their ears in order to smell slightly nice, the rich needed to show off just how rich they were by more conspicuous uses of perfume. It was Otho who induced his friend Emperor Nero to perfume the soles of his feet, an act that has Pliny jumping up and down with rage, 'How pray, could this be noticed, or how could there be any pleasure from that part of the body?'

Elsewhere we find perfume incorporated into architecture: Nero had it squirt from the walls onto his guests and Caligula had his bath tub personally scented. The Emperor Elagabalus employed his own personal perfumer and refused to swim in any pool that had not first been perfumed with saffron. All of which seem harmless (if expensive) eccentricities compared with the fad of Pliny's day, drinking perfume so that your insides smell as sweet as your outside. After that you might decide Pliny had a point after all about wealth bringing about the moral decline of Rome.

Perfumes were available in a multitude of scents, from the simple rosewater to the royal perfume that came from the kings of Parthia and whose ingredients included cinnamon leaves, cypress, lotus, honey and wine. There was balsam, which had to be imported from Judaea, as this was the only place the balsam vine grew. Frankincense was another key ingredient of perfumes, which had to be imported all the way from Arabia where they had to harvest twice a year to keep up with Roman demands.

Which all sound lovely, at least in theory. In practise the application of perfumes was a bit too liberal for some. 'You reek as if a cinnamon flask has been unstoppered and up-ended,' complains Martial, adding the unnecessary final jibe of 'were I to treat my dog the same way, he'd smell just as sweet.'[7] Charming.

Hair

The rule of thumb for hair, which applies to both Roman women and men, was hair on the head was good, hair anywhere else was bad.

Roman women's hairstyles differ according to the era and have become a useful way of dating a bust or statue. Under the Julian Claudian emperors (Augustus, Tiberius, Caligula, Claudius and Nero), the hairstyles of the imperial women move from the very simple bun of Augustus' wife, Livia, to the more elaborate hairstyles of Agrippina and Poppaea, which involved hair plaited across the head with curled ringlets falling onto the neck.

Later styles, such as that sported by Hadrian's sister-in-law, Matidia, were a multitude of plaits woven and curled round into a bun with both tiaras and headbands incorporated into the design (see image 10). In the third century Empress Julia Domna wears her hair waved and loose to her shoulders (see image 11). All these hairstyles we find aped by the population; the imperial ladies were the trendsetters of their day.

There is one period that deserves a special mention for it was here, under the Flavian dynasty (69–96 CE), that Roman lady hairstyles reached their peak: quite literally. The Flavian lady hairdo consisted of a huge looming tower of curls at the front, with a plaited bun at the back. And when I say tower, I mean tower; these frontal additions could be a foot in height. This was the era when hair got BIG (see image 9).

Nobody is entirely sure how these hairstyles were accomplished.[8] They may have been the result of some fierce backcombing, meaning those pristine and perfectly formed curls depicted on busts at the time are very idealised, or they may have been a hairpiece sewn into place. Nobody really knows.

But what we do know is that this was not a hairdo you could achieve by yourself, you needed help. This help came in the shape of a specialist hairdresser known as an Ornatrix. Ornatrices were slaves, but highly skilled ones, and thus competitively expensive. Expensive and skilled they might have been, but that doesn't mean they were treated well. Juvenal describes an overbearing mistress punishing an ornatrix for a single curl being out of place in her Flavian hairdo, the slave suffers the indignity of having her own hair pulled out. Ovid entreats women not to bully their hairdressers by pinching and scratching them, which shows both the poor treatment of slaves in Rome and the stresses for women in having the perfect hairstyle.

Aside from curling, produced by the heating of metal rods to curl the hair around (much like today) and elaborate plaiting affairs, women also had the choice of dying their hair. Henna was in popular use as a hair dye, as well as combinations of berries and nut shells. But the oddest had to be the potion for producing black hair, which was made from leeches mixed with vinegar fermented for several months before being applied.

Just as women dyed their hair, so did men, which invokes mocking. As Martial snidely remarks, 'you were a swan: now you're a crow. You can't fool everyone.'[9]

There was another option if you couldn't stomach having your hair dipped in squelching leech juice, hairpieces and wigs were available. These could be imported from the region whose hair colour you envied, such as the blonde bombshell look, 'Now Germany will send you captured tresses; a conquered nation's gift will save the day!'[10]

With women putting in such time, effort and money into their hair, you might expect their menfolk to at least show a bit of appreciation, but alas no. Ovid bemoans at length about his mistress dying her hair and ruining it, as he sees it, with curling tongs. Juvenal is also brutally rude about those fabulous Flavian lady hairdos, claiming that the effect is absurd. He clearly knows nothing.

The affliction of baldness

Roman women weren't the only ones obsessed with hair care; the men were in on it too. The Emperor Domitian even wrote a book on the subject called *On Care of Hair*. A work Domitian had cause to lament when he began to lose his own hair. The phrasing Suetonius uses on this subject is telling; he refers to 'the disfigurement of baldness'. This same word pops up in Suetonius' description of Julius Caesar. This 'disfigurement' was something his enemies used against him, Suetonius says.

Caesar had his own way of dealing with baldness; he invented the comb over, brushing forward his remaining thin strands of hair over the front of his head. He also became so enormously successful that the Senate voted him the honour of wearing a laurel wreath; a handy covering to disguise his naked head.

The Emperor Otho took this one stage further by having a toupée designed to cover up his baldness. Suetonius claims this wig was so well fashioned that nobody knew of it. A claim that is completely undone by Suetonius writing about it more than seventy years later, and by Otho's own busts and coins on which the hairpiece is laughingly obvious.

Caligula's attempts to disguise his baldness were more authoritarian. He made it a punishable offence for anyone to look down upon him, which had to be stressful for those unnecessarily tall Romans.

Hair was a very sensitive business for men, which possibly explains the presence of terracotta votive hair found at the temple of Asclepius on the Greek island of Kos. If you're thinking it's a little over the top to travel all the way to Kos, a journey that would take at least twelve days[11] involving multiple forms of transport, to ask the healing god to sort out your bald patch, we have testimony that this is exactly what happened. On mainland Greece, in the Temple of Asclepius at Epidaurus, those who had benefited from the healing powers of the god left little messages of thanks, such as this one: 'This man had no hair on his head but lots on his chin. He slept here because he was ashamed at being mocked by other people. By smearing his head with a medicine the god made it have hair.'

Losing your hair was a medical complaint that makes it into the works of Galen and the Hippocratic writings. Their understanding of baldness was based on the humours model of medicine, where humankind was thought to be made up of four substances: blood, yellow bile, black bile and phlegm. These had varying degrees of warmness, dryness, wetness and coldness. A healthy body had an equal amount of these humours: an imbalance of any of them was what led to illness.

For Galen, baldness was caused by too much wet and cold, but also conversely by the dryness of the skin beneath the scalp. The doctors of the Hippocratic writings have a different explanation, hair needs moisture, bald men have a particularly phlegmatic constitution and during sexual intercourse the phlegm in their scalp is heated and agitated, which causes the hair to fall out. Therefore, they go onto explain, eunuchs do not become bald because they do not experience the necessary violent motion of intercourse. Similarly, women during intercourse do not experience as great an agitation as men and that is why they don't go bald either.

Rather than being something that just happened to men at a certain age, baldness was understood as an illness, the physical results of which were just as disfiguring as the itchy skin disease the Emperor Tiberius was said to suffer from. This goes some way to explaining why those Roman emperors mentioned earlier were quite so sensitive about their hair loss and why men were desperate enough to appeal to the gods for help with their affliction. But fear not, for Pliny the Elder has a sure-fire cure for baldness, an ointment of bear grease, laudanum and maidenhair. One can only presume it smelt somewhat.

Body hair

'No rankness of the wild goat under your armpits, no legs bristling with harsh hair!'[12]

If hair on the head was good, hair on the body had a more ambiguous status in ancient Rome. There were several options for removing body hair available to both Roman women and men. If you are sensitive to pain (and let's face it, who isn't) you might want to avoid the plucker. These sadists could be found practising their skills at the baths and making their victims, sorry clients, scream in agony. Something that Seneca complains about when he purchases an apartment over the public baths, alongside the shrill voice of the plucker drumming up business, which both disturb his peace.

Another method of hair removal was the application of heated walnut shells to the area to singe off the hair, which hardly sounds any less painful than plucking. Resins appear to have been used a bit like wax, waiting until they hardened and then ripped off – still not a painless method. Or perhaps, finally, why not just pumice stone the hairs off. Time consuming and presumably not that effective, it will at least leave your eyes tear-free and your skin in one piece.

For women, hair removal was just about acceptable, although there is some sneering to be found in our sources. Martial is spectacularly rude about older women removing their pubic hair, 'Remember what the wise man said, "Don't pluck the lion's beard when he's dead."'[13] Which is just mean.

Pliny the Elder has a similar aversion to the full Brazilian. 'Women's pudenda exposed for all the world to see thanks to depilatories,'[14] he declares. There's an intriguing question here on where on earth Pliny is hanging out that exposes him to quite so many exposed vulvae. Most likely the public baths during mixed bathing sessions.

Removing body hair for men was a bit more contentious. Although excessive body hair was undesirable and likely to get you nicknamed 'goat' (another one of Caligula's enforced rules was the banning of mentioning goats in his presence as it reminded him of his own hairiness) the Romans couldn't get over the fact that all this plucking of body hair might be a bit effeminate. As shown in this particularly filthy Martial epigram:

> Chrestus, your balls are depilated
> And your cock is as smooth as a vulture's neck.
> Your scalp is slicker than a hooker's butt
> And there isn't a bit of stubble on your legs.
> Relentless tweezers have plucked your pale lips clean.[15]

Martial then goes onto to criticise Chrestus for succumbing to the plucker while praising the virtues of Rome's hairy republican ancestors. We are back to that mythical golden age, an age that now includes being hairy; or rather not caring about your appearance. Ovid takes a similar line, suggesting an unkempt beauty is acceptable in a man and the pumice stoning should be left to the Cybele's eunuch priests.

A male obsession with his appearance was not considered properly Roman. Roman men should be concerned with public life, politics and duty, not skincare, hair dye and sorting out a hairy bum. This is very evident in accounts of the Emperor Otho.

The dandy that died well

We met Otho earlier showing Nero how to perfume his feet, but there was more to Otho than nice smelling insoles. He had a sure-fire way of preventing beard growth, a moist bread poultice applied to his cheeks and chin. He also wore a toupée and had plucked out all his body hair.

This care of his body and appearance taints Otho's character as soft and self-obsessed. Juvenal describes a mirror as Otho's constant companion, sneering that he checked his reflection to gaze upon his armour before riding into battle. He is seen as unmanly, which is why his end comes as a surprise to everyone.

Hopelessly outnumbered by Vitellius' forces, Otho elects to commit suicide rather than sacrifice more men to his cause. This very Roman death is commended by all, not least because nobody thought that Otho had such a gesture in him. As Suetonius says, 'I am inclined to think that it was because of these habits that a death so little in harmony with his life excited the greater marvel.'[16] Real proper Roman men did not soften their faces with bread or wear perfume. Any that did were suspect.

If Otho was unmanly for plucking out his body hair, the emperor Elagabalus takes the unmanliness to the next level. Not only did he remove his own body hair, he also rubbed a depilatory ointment on women at the public baths and shaved the groins of his servants personally! With the added yuck factor of then using the same razor to remove his own beard.

Like every other aspect of life for the Roman man, body hair was a balancing act. Too much and you were a hairy barbarian, too little and you risked your manhood being questioned.

A short history of beards

As we saw in an earlier chapter, beards had an important role in the transition of a Roman boy into a man. However, beards were also worn for fashionable purposes.

Beards pop in and out of favour over the history of ancient Rome. The first period of beard popularity is during that mythical golden age, when men were men and far too busy besting foreigners to bother with shaving or any other form of barbering. We know this because Pliny the Elder tells us that the first barber did not arrive in Rome until 300 BCE. Before then, Pliny sagely tells us, Romans did not cut their hair, which offers up all manner of interesting questions and a mental image of Cincinnatus with a man bun.

As for regular shaving, this, Pliny tells us, was introduced to Rome in the second century BCE by a relative of Scipio Africanus who was the first to shave every day. This was revolutionary because prior to that it appears only men over the age of forty shaved. From this point on being clean shaven becomes the norm.

Shaving, and other forms of grooming, become the mark of being a civilised man. We see this play out at times of extreme mental anguish for the individual; for example, when General Varus was killed along with three legions in an ambush by German tribes, Augustus was so distraught we are told he didn't cut his hair or his beard for several months. He would bash his head against the walls of the palace declaring, 'Varus, give me back my legions!' On the death of his beloved sister, Drusilla, Caligula too was demented with grief, and just like Augustus, neglected his grooming, forgetting to cut his hair or shave off his beard.

One of the many reasons Suetonius finds to criticise Nero is that he does not take care of his appearance at all. Nero, Suetonius tell us, let his hair grow long (insert disapproving tut here) and often appeared in public in a dining robe, slippers and with a handkerchief tied round his neck (the latter I am interpreting as a cravat and the dining robe as a house coat, confirming Nero's artistic tastes and style).

During the late Republican period the trimmed beard becomes fashionable with the smart, elite set, or as Cicero delightfully calls them, 'dandies with their chin-tufts,'[17] a charge from which there really is no comeback. After which, aside from Nero's horrific neck beard (Google it if you dare), the smooth, shaved chin maintains its hold over the Roman man until into the second century. Enter probably the most famous Roman beard owner of all, the Emperor Hadrian.

Hadrian probably didn't mean to start a fashion trend. Apparently, he only grew one to hide certain blemishes on his face, but as the most depicted man in the empire, it was inevitably that others would copy his example. The wearing of a beard was no longer uncouth, nor a mark of being uncivilised, but an expectation. We are told that Hadrian refused to make any man a tribune who did not possess a full beard. It is hardly surprising that every career-minded man in Rome immediately sacked their barber and concentrated their efforts on growing enough face fuzz to satisfy the emperor.

After Hadrian followed other bearded emperors, Antoninus Pius, Marcus Aurelius, Commodus and the one with the greatest beard of all time, Lucius Verus. Verus was co-emperor with Marcus Aurelius and statues of him display the glossiest, curliest, and most splendid example of Roman beardedness in all of history. The historian Augusta describes it as almost barbarian in style and adds that, to improve his blonde locks Verus would sprinkle his hair with gold dust. By hair, I am including chin hair in this. Yes, Verus had a sparkling, golden beard. Colour me impressed.

Clothes

There were three garments that made up a Roman woman's attire: the tunic, the *stola* and the *palla*. The tunic consisted of a tube-shaped material fixed at the shoulders with buttons or clasps. Over the top of the ankle-length tunic was the *stola*, or outer dress. The *stola* could have sleeves or not, for winter it might be made of wool and for summer a linen version could be worn.

The *stola* was firmly entrenched in the mind of Romans with respectability and moral decency. Prostitutes, for example, were banned from wearing the *stola* and falling foul of morality laws could strip you of your right to wear it. The final layer of female clothing was the *palla*, or shawl. A rectangular piece of cloth, these could be draped around the body or head, however the woman fancied.

The benefits of the three layers, aside from warmth and decency, was that women could mix different colours together. This you can see in all their vibrancy on the frescos of Pompeii, Herculaneum and elsewhere.

Our (male) writers are infuriatingly silent on what fabulous dresses Roman ladies selected to wear to that extremely fashionable dinner party/ imperial banquet. We hear nothing about the particular style selections of imperial women like Livia or Agrippina. It's almost as if they don't care about women's fashion styles.

There was scope to make an impact fashion wise with the material. Wool, linen and cotton were everyday fabrics; if you wanted to get noticed silk would certainly do that, it was considered luxurious and decadent. It's also another one of those things that really upsets Pliny the Elder, who complains, 'Even men have not been ashamed to adopt silk clothing in summer because of its lightness.'[18] A small slither of hope for Pliny is that men have not yet taken up Assyrian silk dresses, 'so far,' he adds, while presumably crossing his fingers.

Another light material was chiffon, which had the added bonus of being suggestively transparent too. A similar effect could be created with muslin, which Pliny recounts being used in the diaphanous clothes in which women in his day show off.

Of course this kind of material is not entirely proper, as Horace spells out in a passage comparing choosing a wife versus choosing a prostitute:

> A dress-hem down to her ankles, a robe on top,
> A thousand things that stop you gaining an open view.
> With the other type, no problem: You can see her almost
> naked in Coan silk.[19]

The staple of Roman men's clothing was the tunic. Togas were ceremonial clothing and rarely worn outside of politics and religious festivals. Although the tunic was quite a basic garment, men did accessorise to stand out and, obviously, show off. In the fourth century tunics with animal figures on apparently become fashionable, these are teamed up with cloaks made of such a light material that they would blow in the breeze. Although the sceptical Ammianus Marcellinus believes these fashion victims are wafting about their cloaks deliberately to show off the expensive tunics beneath.

Cloaks were another garment that could be used to show off. Caligula's friend Ptolemy showed up at the games in a purple cloak of such eye-catching splendour that the emperor was forced to have him executed. A friend of Martial's paid a shocking 10,000 sesterces for a purple cloak.

Why the obsession with purple? Because, of course, it was the most expensive colour to produce. Purple was produced from sea snails, known as murex, and the most fashionable shade of it came from Tyre.[20] The stripes that denoted that someone was in the senatorial or equestrian class were Tyrian purple and triumphal robes were Tyrian purple mixed in with gold. But by Pliny the Elder's day purple had moved from the ceremonial to the everyday. He is aghast that purple is so commonplace that most houses were possessed of purple dining couches.

The most extravagantly and fashionably dressed men in Rome were, naturally, the emperors and we have descriptions of some stonking attire worn by their imperial majesties. Commodus, for example, attended the games in a silk ankle-length tunic woven with gold before changing into a purple robe with golden spangles on. Caligula favoured embroidered cloaks studded with precious gems and (Pliny the Elder look away now!) silk tunics. Elagabalus ups the ante by being the first man in Rome to wear only silk garments, saying that linen was for beggars.

What is beauty?

We have looked at the ways both men and women used make up, perfume, hair and clothes to enhance their attractiveness. But what did the Romans consider attractive? What made a woman beautiful or a man handsome?

Surprisingly, there is scant mention of what a beautiful woman should look like, even in love poetry, where we might expect to find gushing descriptions of their great love, there is very little. Reading through Catullus' entire output will leave you none the wiser as to what Lesbia looked like in any detail. There is mention of black eyes, a pretty foot, a small nose and long fingers, which is hardly enough to sketch a picture from.

Elsewhere Catullus lists the individual attributes of a certain Quintia as being attractive: she is fair, tall and of good posture. Again, rather scant on details and certainly not nearly enough to understand why Quintia is considered a beauty in Rome.

Thankfully, Ovid gives us a bit of detail about what he finds attractive in his mistress, Corinna; her white neck, smooth belly, high breasts and long waist. Although Ovid's taste in women is somewhat liberal, as he himself admits, 'The looks that lure my love have no set pattern.'[21] He likes blondes, he likes the auburn haired, he likes those with dark locks or sable. He likes tall girls or is it short? He likes a ripe youth or a mature lady. He'll even snuggle up with a critic of his poems! Or, you know, a total fan girl. You get the picture.

Martial is very clear on what he likes in a lady, not too skinny but not too fat. Or as he, charmingly puts it: 'Good meat, not blubber on my plate.'[22] Martial's ideal woman is 'a wife who's true to you and yet no prude in bed.'[23]

Horace gives us some clues on what might be attractive by telling us what isn't. 'Oh, what legs, what arms! True, but she's narrow-hipped, long-nosed: short waist, big feet.'[24] From which we may deduce that wide-hipped, short-nosed, long waist and small feet are the things to avoid.

The picture is no clearer for men, with the added disadvantage that we simply don't have the female voices to tell us what they found attractive in a man. Lucius Verus was certainly popular with the ladies, but whether that was down to his fabulous beard or his status as being an enormously powerful man with unlimited wealth, we can't answer.

Tacitus describes a certain Caecina as young, good-looking and tall, without any qualification as to what made Caecina good looking. Fascinatingly, Caecina, despite being fully Roman and only having been in Germania for a couple of years maximum, goes completely native and starts wearing patterned trousers and a plaid cloak. Perhaps that raw barbarian-esque quality was what made him good-looking?

Lucian sums up the ideally attractive man as one who works hard to achieve a body that is neither skinny nor fat. One who has both strength and stamina. One in possession of a tanned face and a fiery spirit of manliness. The message is clear: the perfect male body, just like the perfect male character, takes hard work and dedication. It's all very Roman.

We may glean a little of what was considered at least attractive, if not necessarily sexy, in a man from the work of the doctor Soranus. In his chapter on caring for new-borns he suggests that the baby's nurse massage the child's parts for them to be of a pleasing shape in adulthood. From his description we may deduce that a straight spine, rounded buttocks, a head that is neither too long nor too pointy, smooth kneecaps and not having an aquiline nose are all desirable traits of the Roman male.

Peeking beneath the stola and the toga

No tour of what made Roman men and women sexy would be complete without looking at those parts involved in sexual intercourse. We have talked a bit about 'down there' earlier when we discussed whether hair removal meant the full Brazilian (concluding that yes it did) but now let us dip a bit lower (both physically and tastefully) and look at the aesthetics of genitalia.

Men

Time to discuss penises, because the Romans certainly did and scrawled pictures of them on every possible surface. These penises were most likely a symbol of good luck or perhaps not – nobody thought to helpfully leave an explanation beside their penis graffiti (for which we curse them). We will talk about the multitude of ancient dick pics in a later chapter and what they mean, but here let us talk about the specifics of a good penis.

Thoughts on what made the perfect Roman penis started young. Soranus, in his inspection of a new-born baby boy, is very clear that foreskins are a good thing. To ensure an adult Roman male has a decent one his nurse, post baby bath, should take care to pull his foreskin down so that it covers the entire penis. Should there be difficulty with its length she is advised to secure it down with a piece of wool. As an aside she should also shape the scrotum.

That foreskins were standard for Roman males is backed up by events that occurred during Domitian's reign. The emperor had imposed a tax on Rome's Jewish population, and being ever thorough, this was levied not only on those who practised their religion but those who didn't. This led to some unpleasant scenes, which the biographer Suetonius personally witnessed, of elderly men being stripped and examined before the court to see if they were circumcised.

Circumcision, although allowed for those of the Jewish faith,[25] was considered on a par with castration for Roman citizens and treated as such in the law from the time of Antonius Pius (in the second century CE). The penalties for being involved in an act of circumcision were alarmingly harsh. Romans who allowed themselves or their slaves to be circumcised had their property confiscated and were exiled to an island for life, and any doctors involved were put to death.

Given the Roman love of the baths and communal toilets, circumcision was not something that could escape notice. These harsh laws perhaps explain Soranus' obsession with ensuring a male Roman had a full-length foreskin from the very day he was born.

When we think of Roman art, particularly Roman nude art, what comes to mind is those white, marble statues with their chiselled torsos, firm thighs, squeezable buttocks, and if we are lucky, surviving diddly penises. Small penises are the norm on statues, whether they be representations of gods or emperors. This would suggest that the ideal Roman penis, the penis every Roman male should aspire to possess nestling in their loin cloths, was a neatly compact one.

However, there are exceptions to this penis rule where we find depicted a *sopio*, that is a grossly enlarged penis. The most famous owner of a *sopio* is the god Priapus. Priapus as a subject for art has been raising the eyebrows of visitors to Pompeii for generations. He is the subject of several frescos and some really quite eye-opening (and possibly eye poking) statues. Gosh, is all I can say. You will be unsurprised to learn that Priapus is the god of fertility, as well as a protector of livestock, plants and gardens. The latter of which is a traditional location for a statue of the god.

Priapus is the subject of a collection of explicit epigrams. These short poems were fixed to the base of the god's statue and they demonstrate the protective nature of Priapus. By protective, I mean threatening indignities against anyone who dares to violate the garden or household of Priapus' domain, 'Thou shalt be buggered (lad!), thou also (lass!) shalt be rogered; While for the bearded thief is the third penalty kept.'[26]

Yes, we are back to those Roman threats of sexual violence. The third punishment kept for the thief is of course *irrumo*, oral rape, which appears again and again: robbers will be, 'Sodomised with my twelve-inch phallus. But if so severe and unpleasant a punishment shall not avail, I will strike higher.'[27]

However, Priapus' engrossed member is not just a weapon of violence. Elsewhere in this collection of poems we find the repeated theme that these statues of Priapus are providing fun for the local women, 'Hither! ye Romans! Either lop off my seminal member, which the neighbouring women, ever itching with desire, exhaust the whole night through –more lecherous than sparrows in the spring – or I shall be ruptured.'[28]

Which begs us to ask the question; did size matter? As we have seen in previous chapters the Romans weren't half judgmental and so it should not surprise us that not only were they super competitive on matters of behaviour and character, but also on bodily matters. One place where you could check out your rival's bits was of course that hotbed of iniquity, the baths.

It is from accounts of eyeballing here that we can say that size certainly mattered for some Romans. Ones such as Hostius Quadra, a man so vile and depraved that when he was murdered by his own attendants Augustus weighed it up and decided that, contrary to the law, Quadra's slaves should not all be executed for his death because he wasn't worth avenging. This is quite something given Augustus' adherence to traditional values.

Seneca has quite the detail on what made Quadra so uniquely vile. One such reason he gives is Quadra's obsession with large penises. 'In all the public baths he would recruit favourites and chose men by their obvious size.'[29] So obsessed by size was Quadra that he had mirrors constructed that magnified the reflection, so that he might enjoy looking at an exaggerated form of his partners' penis while they were buggering him.

Quadra isn't the only one sizing men up at the baths. Apparently, it was a bit of a spectator sport, or so Martial would have us believe. 'If from the baths you hear a round of applause, Maron's giant prick is bound to be the cause.'[30] The baths in Martial's time are frequented by their very own Hostius Quadra, Cotta. Although Cotta is using penis size to decide who he should invite to his dinner parties, Martial's tackle does not meet Cotta's standards, much to his irritation.

Emperor Elagabalus, like Quadra, was another one of the firm belief that bigger is better. He had certainly worked out the priorities of the job and we are told 'did nothing but send out agents to search for those who had particularly large organs and bring them to the palace in order that he might enjoy their vigour.'[31]

Both Quadra and Elagabalus are presented as the very worst, most depraved of men and their obsession with big penises is firmly tied to their sexual deviances. They like big penises because they are submitting to anal sex, a most un-Roman position.

Aside from Priapus, we find satyrs, the hairy legged half-goat acolytes of Bacchus depicted with overly large, erect penises. These fellows pop up on vases from ancient Greece and are up to all manner of shenanigans, whether it be balancing wine craters on their erection, attempting sex with a wine skin or having sex with one another. Satyrs are comic relief, and their penises play a role in that, the permanent erection denoting a constant lust that leads them to unseemly actions such as propositioning a goat.

We are back to that Roman notion of not being excessive in anything you do, including sex, a lesson the satyrs have not learned, making them both ridiculous and open to public ridicule. A hugely oversized erect penis was unsavoury and unseemly and hinted at a defective moral character; *virtus* light in other words.

We will leave the final word on the subject to Greek comic playwright, Aristophanes, who states what makes the ideal male body, 'a gleaming chest, bright skin, broad shoulders, tiny tongue, strong buttocks, and a little prick.'[32]

Women

We've discussed in our previous chapters the patriarchal nature of Roman society, the male obsession with their penises and where they are going to put them to come out on top in a highly competitive world. We've discussed how laws were made in relation to the mutilation of male genitalia, such as circumcision and castration. In a later chapter we will examine the ubiquitous image of the phallus, which was depicted everywhere in ancient Rome. With all this light shone on what was between male legs, you will be unsurprised to learn that not nearly the same attention is given to what the ladies had on offer.

Vaginas, although they make it into medical texts, are rarely referred to elsewhere in literature, and when they are, it is not as an erotic ideal or a preference but rather as something that disgusts. Think back to Martial's poem on grey pubic hair. Although, if you thought that poem was mean, then you might want to downgrade that thought, because there's worse to come on Martial's take on vaginas. Brace yourself.

Martial starts his poem on the subject, with the line 'Lydia is as wide as the ass of a bronze rider's horse,'[33] and really it's downhill from there as he compares more 'roomy' items to Lydia's vagina. These include the trousers of a British pauper and the throat of a pelican, which are images you really don't want conjured in your mind. He concludes horribly with this: 'I am reputed to have fucked her in a salty fishpond. I am not sure: I think I fucked the fishpond.'

I'm afraid we are not done with Martial's vagina complaints, there's also this about his lady friend, Galla: 'Whenever I came to you and we were moved about with mingling groins, you were silent – but your vagina wasn't.'[34] Yes, as well as loose vaginas Martial has a problem with noisy ones: 'Who can laugh at the little pops of a garrulous pussy? When it makes it sound, whose penis does not fall with his desire?'

Martial concludes that he would have much preferred sodomising her, which just about sums up Roman males.

Chapter 7

Finding Love:
Courting on the Streets of Rome

Marriage was considered the acceptable and proper route for all Romans. It was, certainly at the elite end of society, an arranged affair between families. However, sex was certainly not restricted to within marriage, for men at least. But there were restrictions, both legal and cultural. 'Love whatever you want, as long as you stay away from married ladies, widows, virgins, young men and free boys,'[1] says Plautus. We may add to this list, freeborn women.

Freeborn women were appointed a male guardian to oversee their financial affairs (and likely poke their noses into their other business too) and were protected under the laws relating to *stuprum*. This lack of access to freeborn girls is a prominent theme in Roman love poetry. Attracting the love of their lady is the easy part, continuing the liaison is more challenging thanks in part to the door. This door is both a metaphorical barrier to their love and, well, an actual door. As Tibullus complains: 'The harsh door shut fast with a solid bolt.'[2]

Tibullus has a lot of problems with the door, desperately wishing it to open and reveal his mistress, Delia. Lord knows how many hours he spends staring at the door, but he hits that moment of despair familiar to all of us who have waited for a late running train or bus and mentally pleaded 'please god let it come!'

> Door, of a surly master, may the rain beat on you,
> and lightning hurled on Jupiter's orders find you out.
> Door, open now, conquered by my complaints alone.[3]

Propertius is another one troubled by doors, 'Why are your solid doors closed now, and mute, for me?'[4] Suffering dreadfully from shut door syndrome, the poet debates how much easier it would be for him to just take up with prostitutes.

It's an interesting poem because it spells out the difficulties, door aside, of courting the freeborn (without family support, it should be added). Poor Propertius is forced to bribe slaves to take messages to his mistress and wander around Rome trying to locate her. And then finally dish out more of his money to the keeper of that bolted door to see her.

Ovid ups the door suffering with a poem dedicated to his mistress' doorkeeper, 'Look – you can see, then, undo the lock – the doorway's wet with my tears!'[5] Ovid is an enterprising sort, and he finds a way to gain access to his girlfriend that doesn't involve dishing out money, he makes friends with her closest female slave. And by 'friends' we mean he has sex with her.

Although as Horace notes, you might well have to deal with more than one servant in your way.

> If you want what's forbidden (since that is what excites you),
> What walls protect, there's a host of things in your way,
> Bodyguards, closed litters, hairdressers, hangers-on.[6]

Is Ovid prepared to bed the hairdressers and bodyguards too? We're going to say yes; definitely yes.

As well as the physical barrier of the door there were further less wooden impediments to dating the freeborn. Men had their *virtus* to preserve and women had their reputation for chastity. Freeborn women had much to lose from an unwise sexual liaison, or even the rumour of one. Which is not to say they didn't have them, as we saw earlier and will cover again later, but rather that it was more difficult to pursue a sexual relationship with a freeborn woman than women of other status.

Being freeborn, whether you were male or female, was to enjoy exalted rights such as protection under the *stuprum* laws. This, however, may have added to the illicit excitement. Martial has a wry epigram aimed a certain Caecilianus, whose wife nobody fancied until he employed a house guard (the likes of which made Ovid cry), and this produced a crowd of would-be lovers.

If women were so well protected, how did a Roman man go about courting her? Over to Publius Ovid Naso, first century CE poet and famous exile, who we last saw explaining a proper beauty regime. There's more to Ovid than removing armpit hair and the correct amount of rouge on a cheek: he also does a neat line in dating advice, thus proving himself the *Marie Claire* of the ancient world.[7]

In the *Arts of Love*, the poet details his proven method for picking up women (Spoiler Alert: it doesn't involve getting the respective families together to hammer out the dowry arrangements).

Despite those pesky morality laws, and despite societal expectations placed on both sexes, the reality was clearly different. We know women weren't unobtainable objects locked in houses weaving away, untouched by any man who was not their father or husband, for several reasons. One is the very existence of Roman love poetry, or as a Twitter pal of mine once referred to it, 'whining to metre'. Love poetry is a literary genre dedicated to loving a woman, pursing a woman, getting a woman, then regretting getting the woman because she's a bloody nightmare and smashes their sensitive heart beneath her best high-heeled sandals.

Outside of love poetry, witty epigram writer Martial seems to have no problem finding women on the streets of Rome, and serial complainer Juvenal's bitter raging about women would hardly have hit the mark as satire if women were whiling the day away weaving underwear and being dutiful.

We will look in a later chapter of those women who really broke the mould (and the gossip monitor gauge) with some truly scandalous behaviour, but for now let us sit at the knee of uncle Ovid and drink in his pulling techniques. He opens his seduction school with the claim, 'Who in this town knows not the lovers art should read this book and ply on the expert's part.'

Let us reserve judgement on Ovid's 'expertise' until we've heard what he has to say. First up are his top tips for finding the woman of your dreams. He opens with this cracker: 'She won't come falling for you out of thin air: the right girl has to be searched for: use your eyes.'

This is perhaps illuminating on the dimness of the audience he is addressing. He then launches into an extended metaphor about hunting, which is all very noble and stirring, and bound to gee-up the young horny man, but which is instantly undone in the epic grandeur stakes when he titles his next chapter 'Search while you are out walking'. I guess you'll not be needing that javelin and net, Gaius.

We shouldn't be so hard on Ovid, it is not so easy to pick up attractive freeborn women in the same way that is in modern times. Although there are bars and cookshops in Rome aplenty, you are unlikely to meet a woman of Ovid's class frequenting them because they are extremely rough. So rough are these cookshops that emperors periodically shut the whole damn lot of them down to give the urban cohorts a rest from breaking up fights.

So where do you meet women? Ovid has several suggestions in his chapter on walking about the city: the colonnades of Pompey's theatre feature, presumably because you can grab a bit of privacy by grabbing your beloved behind one of the pillars. Also mentioned are the theatre of Marcellus, Livia's portico, the shrine of Adonis and the temple of Isis. Make sure you wear comfy sandals because the walk from the theatres of Pompey and Marcellus to Livia's portico is 1.7km, and it's a further 1.8km from there to the temple of Isis. Which might not seem like much but on a hot day and with Rome being highly overpopulated with lots of people to get in your way, it's going to get tiring fast – and that's before you factor in the effort involved with Ovid's seduction techniques.

Aside from walking about the city hoping to stumble across a beauty, where else does Ovid recommend meeting the fairer sex? The chariot races are a prime opportunity, Ovid tells us, because the benches are set up so close together, meaning the spectators are pressed up against each other. You might want to make sure you are squished next to an attractive lady for the duration.

Once you are settled you are ready to deliver up Ovid's killer opening chat up line, 'Whose team is that?' For this to take maximum effect it must be said earnestly, and one would assume a little stupidly given chariot teams are divided into colours – the reds, greens, blues and whites – and all participants are wearing those colours prominently. Although maybe this is a deliberate ploy to imply innocence and thus lessen the impact of Ovid's next tip: being a full-on sex pest.

You should, Ovid advises, flick an imaginary speck of dust from her bosom. Lift her skirt under the pretext of preventing her hem line getting muddy. Adjust her foot stoll and reposition her cushion, with dexterous touch he says, so let us assume this involves some kind of bum fondling.

Given a single chariot race was seven laps and there might be twenty-four races staged that day, this leaves a considerable amount of time for Ovid's acolytes to press their suit. The result being that if she can stand your attentions for that long without slapping you round the face, then you are probably made for each other.

The Games are another location that Ovid highlights as being a top place for totty gathering.[8] Here, he suggests you give a detailed commentary on the events for your companion, without worrying about how accurate this commentary is. In fact, why not invent the whole thing? This could go either way; it could be a charmingly imaginative tale or bullshit from beginning to end. A lot will depend on your natural charisma, or lack thereof. We'll ignore the patronising assumption that women are unable to understand the proceedings of the amphitheatre on their own.

Other spots recommended for some heavy-duty courting include festivals, chiefly because of the amount of wine involved. Or as Ovid rather charmingly puts it, 'wine lights the fire of passion in the soul, cares melt and vanish in the brimming bowl.' Though you must take care, Ovid warns us, because, 'Your eye for beauty's warped by night and wine.'[9] This surely must be the earliest mention of the mind-bending effects of beer goggles.

The theatre is apparently a top place to secure a lady lover, both keepers or a casual fling, or as our instructor rather creepily puts it, a toy or a lasting joy. The emotion a play induces in the audience is to be taken advantage of, we are told.

Although Ovid might be out of luck because, according to Juvenal, it's the actors the lady audience members want to seduce rather than any fellow audience member. The actors have the advantage of that magical pixie dust of fame, which they clearly worked for all it was worth since Juvenal claims their lady admirers would collect souvenirs of their favourite thespians. So damn sexy are actors that they can cause regrettable bodily functions in their female fans, 'When sinuous Bathyllus dances his pantomime Leda Tucia loses control of her bladder, and Apula yelps, as if she were making love, with sharp tedious cries.'[10]

Aside from hanging about public venues, flicking through your copy of *Arts of Love* and practising saying, 'Whose team is that?' repeatedly to get the level of earnestness just right, there is the opportunity to meet women at your workplace. If you are a lawyer, that is.

Ovid suggests that lawyers use their platform for some heavy workplace flirting by shooting saucy suggestive looks at any attractive women watching their trial. We must hope they do this without getting distracted from pleading their client's case. Although given that speeches in Roman court trials can last up to seven hours at a time, that's an exhausting amount of saucy looks to throw convincingly and non-repetitively.

A more fun suggestion of Ovid's for meeting the ladies is to head to Baiae. This was a super fashionable resort located on what is now the bay of Naples and from other sources it sounds quite marvellous. This is evident from another one of those improving letters from Seneca where he slags it off something rotten, saying, 'We ought to select abodes which are wholesome not only for the body but also for the character.'[11]

Seneca's particular objections to Baiae are that there are people drunkenly wandering about the beaches, 'serenading in the night' (or more probably drunken singing) and boat parties with lewd women. He tells his friend/reluctant pen pal that 'he should choose an austere and pure dwelling-place,' so exactly not what Seneca has done. Although, perhaps Seneca considers his character strong enough to withstand Baiae's temptations and is only repeatedly returning to check that it is as lewd as he remembered.

Baiae had acquired a certain reputation. The saying went that it was the place where old men went to become boys again and boys went to become girls. Martial sardonically says that a visitor to Baiae arrived a Penelope and left a Helen.[12] Baiae's reputation for corrupting even the most innocent of visitors has Propertius in a panic when his on/off/off/on again mistress, Cynthia, takes a holiday there. He despairs that Baiae is fatal to chaste girls, although his Cynthia is not chaste in any way, much to his to his anguish. All of which is encouraging for your chances of pulling there. Don't bother packing a bucket and spade, you'll be far too busy hanging out with those lewd women on board their boats.

To summarise: women can be found in public places, you should sit next to them and strike up conversation by feigning earnest ignorance, or for the more confident spin them an elaborate line of bullshit. Wine and emotion are to your advantage. You should use your proximity to touch them up repeatedly in a way that they can't really complain about. Or else head down to the coast where everybody is permanently pissed and up for it. Good luck!

Outside of Ovid's dubious advice, banquets appear to be a good place to get off with a lady. Octavian certainly pulled successfully at a banquet: it was where he first met his wife of fifty years, Livia. According to scurrilous rumour, spread by Mark Antony, mid banquet Octavian led Livia from the dining room to a bed chamber. She returned with 'her hair in disorder and her ears glowing'.[13] It should be noted that this banquet was being held at the home of Livia and her then husband, Tiberius. He didn't remain her husband for long.

Octavian was not alone in getting carried away at a banquet. Juvenal describes the effect the hired dancing girls induced by their wriggling bottoms, an action that lit the fires of both the men and women watching, he claims.

Imperial banquets naturally have the best opportunities on offer. Nero, for example, offered entertainment that included a selection of wild animals to marvel at, and then, when you'd finished marvelling at the animals, you could head down to the brothels he'd had specially constructed for the party.

If your tastes run in the other direction, then the luxurious banquet that Lucius Verus held might be for you. Generous to a fault, he gave plentiful gifts to his guests, including jewelled cups made from gold, Alexandrine crystals, out of season flowers and 'the comely lads who did the serving were given as presents, one to each guest,'[14] along with the meat carvers so you could recreate the joyous evening at home.

If for some unfathomable reason you didn't move in those types of illustrious circles, you could still meet attractive ladies by securing a job that grants you access to their homes. Having a legitimate reason to be there means you pass straight through the door like a ghost. Being a music teacher seems to be a viable route; Juvenal is certainly convinced they are all having it off with their pupils. But then Juvenal is also convinced that women are all having sex with their eunuchs, which as well as being physically impossible rather dents Juvenal's credibility.

If all this courting sounds quite exhausting, potentially fruitless and possibly likely to get you in trouble with the law then you might prefer just to stay home and get it on with your slave.[15]

Chapter 8

Getting Down to Business: Sex

We have talked about language, had a quick tour through 400 years of morality laws, examined the ideals for men and women both in character and appearance, and discussed how to find a lover. It's time now to get down to business: sexual intercourse.

Having got this far into this book you will be fully aware by now that Romans were not shy about talking about sex, even when the sex was not great, such as poor Pliny the Elder whose love life clearly wasn't all that: 'All other animals derive satisfaction from having mated; man gets almost none.'[1] Therefore, we have plenty of material on what was good sex, what was bad sex and what was unacceptable sex. But let us begin at the beginning with first sex.

First sex, or virginity

'Man is the only animal whose first experience of mating is accompanied by regret.' So says Pliny the Elder, who we have to assume lost his virginity in less than satisfying circumstances before embarking on that lifetime of terrible sex.

The ancient Roman relationship with virginity is very different to what we might find in an equivalent Christian society. Given the amount of divorce and remarriage, virginity certainly wasn't an expected state on entrance to marriage. This held true even for empresses: Livia had been married before Augustus, Agrippina before Claudius, Poppaea before Nero and I could go on.

Also remember all those virtuous women of the golden age: Verginia was a virgin, Lucretia and the Claudia Quinta were married women. Virginity itself was not a recommending quality; chasteness, childbearing and adherence to the values of that mythical golden age was what elevated women.

Discussions of virginity appear in the medical field, and more particularly whether being a virgin was good for your health or not. Intercourse was thought to moisten the uterus, without this moistness the womb would become dry and painful. Pliny the Elder states that intercourse is known to cure pain in the lower regions, as well as impaired vision, soundness of mind and depression.

In his book on gynaecology, Soranus debates the pros and cons of remaining a virgin. There is no moral tone here, Soranus is entirely fixated on whether permanent virginity is good for the body. On the pro side he notes that pregnancy and childbirth exhaust a woman's body, that desire can suck the energy from the body and that those women who have taken up religious roles that require virginity are stronger and less susceptible to diseases.

On the cons side he notes that virgins are not free from desire and can suffer greatly from sexual frustration. Intercourse is also determined to be good at relaxing a woman's body and particularly her uterus, which makes menstruation easier. Virgins, Soranus says, suffer greatly from menstruation problems and backs this up by noting that women who remarry after a long widowhood often start to menstruate more freely.

Soranus doesn't really come down firmly on one side or the other but makes a case that some virgins will suffer from their state, while others will be strengthened by it. As for the right age for a woman to lose her virginity, Soranus is clear: whatever her desires, a girl should wait until her periods start before being deflowered. Soranus notes this is around fourteen years of age and designates this is the best age, with a warning that waiting too long to lose your virginity can be harmful to your health. The minimum age for marriage, determined by Augustus, was twelve for girls and fourteen for boys. Most girls married for the first time between the ages of twelve and fifteen, which holds with Soranus' recommendation.

Interestingly, Soranus in his discussion on virginity does not believe there is such a thing as a hymen, 'For it is a mistake to assume that a thin membrane grows across the vagina dividing it and this membrane causes pain when burst in defloration.'[2] Rather, Soranus believes that the vagina in virgins contains furrows and vessels which burst when spread apart during that first act of intercourse.

Good sex

As we have seen in the section on virginity, intercourse was considered good for the health and might even be prescribed by a doctor. A case is mentioned in medical texts of an ailing woman whose illness the doctors agreed was caused by her long widowhood. Their prescription was for her to marry quickly and presumably have sex morning, noon and night. Sex, therefore, is good for all manner of ailments and complaints, but nowhere does it state whether this medicinal intercourse needs to be of a certain quality for the cure to work.

In Rome sex was not something that was hidden away and not talked about, it was very much in the public discourse and that public discourse included what was good sex. But firstly, let us head back to our pal Martial, who is quite happy to complain at length on what he doesn't like in bed.

I will spare you all his whinging and summarise his thoughts on the subject. This is what Martial dislikes in sex: being told to hold back on his climax, being called mouse or precious lover, overly aggressive hand jobs, motionless sexual partners and partners that refuse anal sex.[3] He does dedicate a whole poem to how annoying he finds the noise of his partner's vagina, so we will add that to his list of dislikes. Ultimately, what Martial likes are uninhabited sexual partners who will perform the acts he likes.

There's plenty of material for what the Romans considered good sex in Ovid's other work on Love, the *Amores,* in which where he dishes out sex tips for both men and women. There is little in Ovid on discussing the merits of various sexual positions, the nearest we get is his suggestion for women that they choose a position that flatters their assets. Top tip from Ovid for those with flabby post-childbirth tummies: take it from behind.

> What is interesting is the emphasis on mutual pleasure:
> Don't let modesty prevent you touching her.
> You'll see her eyes flickering with tremulous brightness,
> as sunlight often flashes from running water.
> Moans and loving murmurs will arise,
> and sweet sighs, and playful and fitting words.[4]

He stresses that the lover should take his time and not rush things. In such an aggressively male society we perhaps would not expect there to be much consideration given to the woman's pleasure in love making, yet here is Ovid giving ample lines to the subject of female orgasm as a desirable part of sex. For Ovid sex is a partnership, 'that's the fullness of pleasure, when man and woman lie there equally spent.'

That women enjoyed sex is also mentioned in the Hippocratic writings, it is noted that once sex begins the woman feels pleasure until the man ejaculates and that she can also climax, experiencing an orgasm. Soranus is of the mind that women more readily conceive if they have the appetite for sex, or as we would say, they are feeling horny.

The Hippocratic writers are very clear that men enjoy sex more due to their role in it being more vigorous, but grant that the woman's pleasure lasts longer. However, elsewhere we find a lingering view that women enjoy sex more than men, not least in the story of Tiresias.

The best of both worlds: Tiresias

The king of the gods, Jupiter, was embroiled in an argument with his wife, Juno, over whether men or women enjoy sex more. Jupiter was convinced that women did but Juno denied this vehemently. To settle the argument, they called for Tiresias. Why Tiresias? Because he had lived and loved as both a man and a woman, and so was uniquely qualified to answer their question.

Tiresias' sex change had come about suddenly. One day he had stumbled across two snakes copulating, which, for reasons obscure, enraged him horribly. He beat at the snakes with a stick, which in turn enraged the goddess Juno and as a punishment she turned him into a woman. Tiresias spent seven years living as a woman and even popped out a few children during that time.

Having successfully mastered being a woman, Tiresias again stumbled across two snakes having a sexy time, but this time he did not beat them with a stick but rather let them be and was turned back into a man.[5]

Mythology is awash with morals such as not getting too big for your boots (hubris), not believing yourself to be equal to the gods (arrogance) and not sleeping with Jupiter (stupid). To which we can add, snakes are entitled to a sex life so leave them alone.

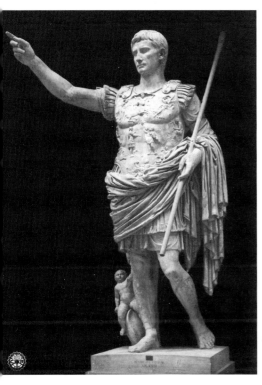

1. Rome's greatest morality master, the emperor Augustus. (*Wellcome Collection, Photographic postcard, public domain*)

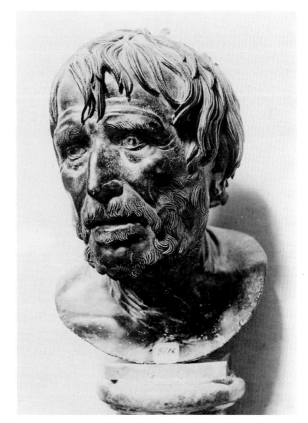

Stoic philosopher and tutor to Nero,
Seneca. (*Wellcome Collection. Attribution
0 International* (*CC BY 4.0*))

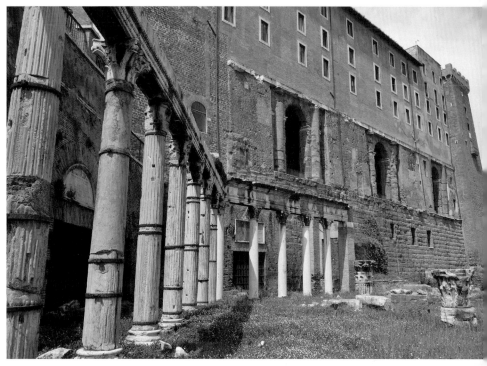

3. The Tabularium on the Capitol Hill in Rome, where new citizens of the city were registere (*Graham Ferguson/Shutterstock*)

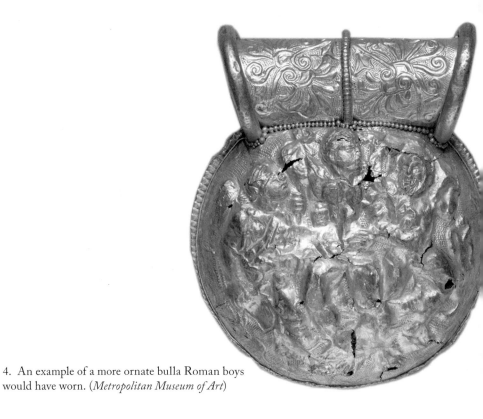

4. An example of a more ornate bulla Roman boys would have worn. (*Metropolitan Museum of Art*)

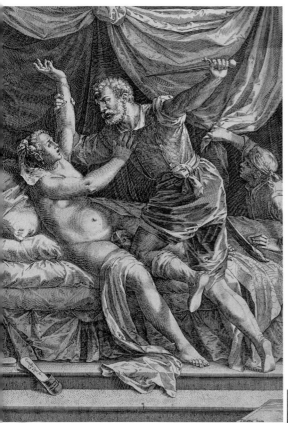

5. A 16th century representation of the rape of Lucretia that brought down the Roman monarchy. (*Line engraving by C. Cort after Titian, 1571. Wellcome Collection. Attribution 4.0 International (CC BY 4.0)*)

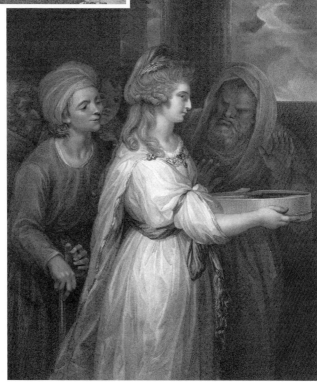

The Vestal Virgin Tuccia being ~~in~~spected while carrying water in a ~~sie~~ve to prove her chastity. (*Etching ~~by~~ P.W. Tomkins, 1798, after Sir ~~J. R~~eynolds, Wellcome Collection. ~~At~~tribution 4.0 International ~~(C~~C BY 4.0)*)

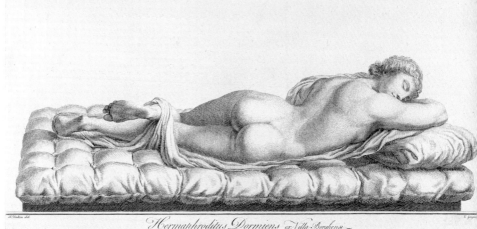

7. The Sleeping Hermaphroditus. (*Etching by C. Grignion after R. Dalton, 1744, Wellcome Collect Attribution 4.0 International (CC BY 4.0)*)

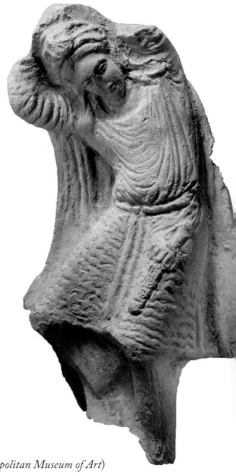

8. Terracotta statuette of a dancing youth. (*Metropolitan Museum of Art*)

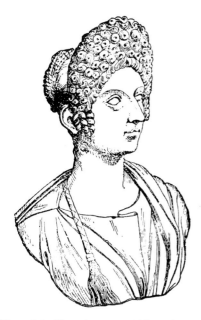

Flavia Julia Titi, daughter of Titus. (*Vintage*
aved illustration. Morphant Creation/
tterstock)

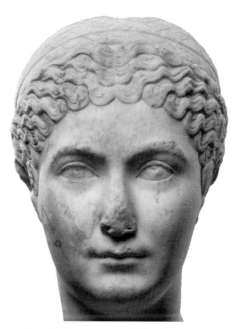

10. Marble portrait of Matidia.
(*Metropolitan Museum of Art*)

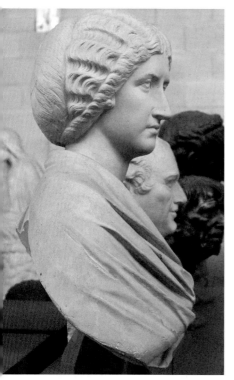

Julia Domna, wife to Septimius Severus,
rting her do. (*Museum of Classical Archaeology,*
nbridge no.537. (Original: Rome, Capitoline
seums, inv. no. 280))

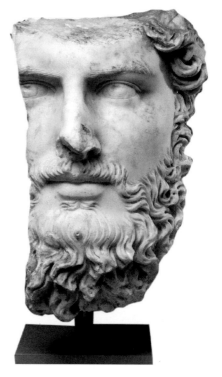

12. Marble portrait of the co-emperor
Lucius Verus. (*Metropolitan Museum of Art*)

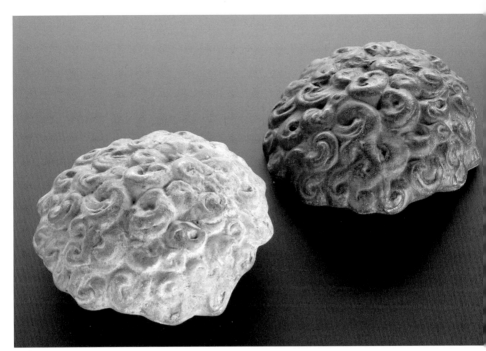

13. Terracotta votive scalp, Roman, 200 BCE–200 CE. (*Science Museum, London. Attribution International (CC BY 4.0)*)

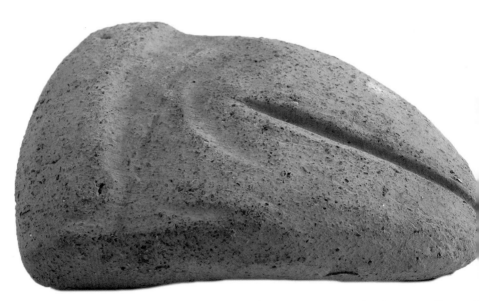

14. A clay-baked vulva. Roman votive offering. (*Wellcome Collection. Attribution 4.0 Internati (CC BY 4.0)*)

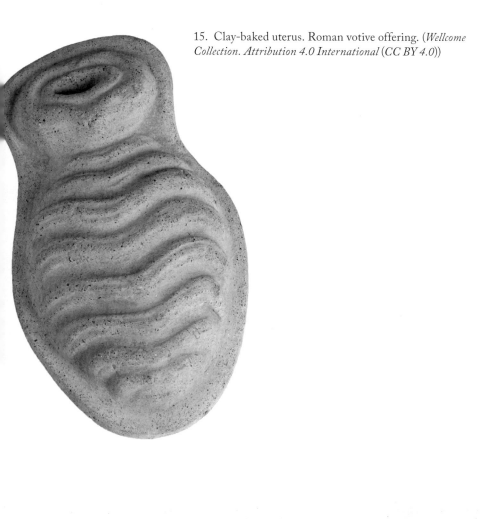

15. Clay-baked uterus. Roman votive offering. (*Wellcome Collection. Attribution 4.0 International* (*CC BY 4.0*))

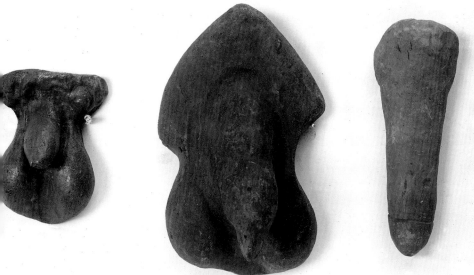

16. Three Roman votive offerings: penis. (*Wellcome Collection. Attribution 4.0 International* (*CC BY 4.0*))

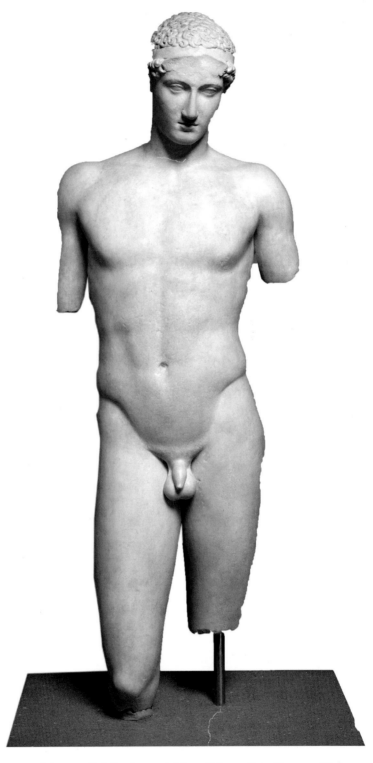

17. Marble statue of the so-called Stephanos Athlete. (*Metropolitan Museum of Art*)

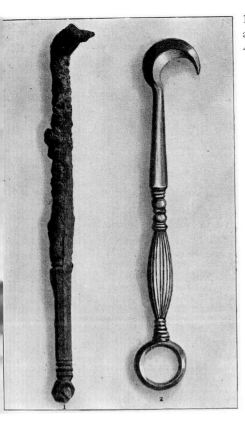

18. Roman surgical instruments, embryo hook and decapitator. (*Wellcome Collection. Attribution 4.0 International* (*CC BY 4.0*))

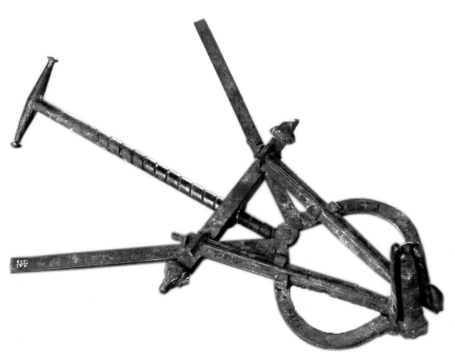

19. Copy of vaginal speculum, Europe, 1901–1939. (*Wellcome Collection, Attribution 4.0 International* (*CC BY 4.0*))

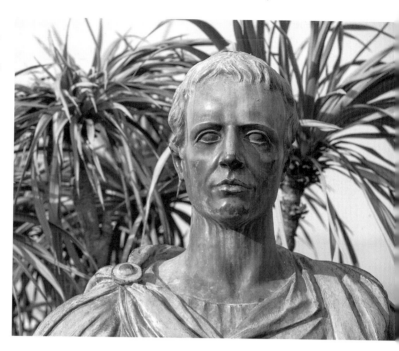

20. Statue of the roman poet Gaius Valerius Catullus in Sirmione, Lake Garda, Italy. (*Shutterstock*)

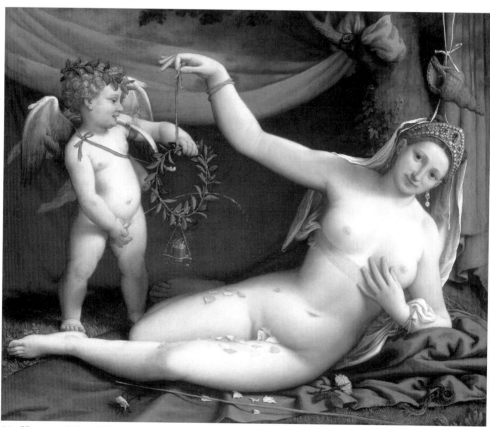

21. Venus and Cupid Lorenzo Lotto (Italian, Venice ca. 1480–1556 Loreto). (*Courtesy of Metropolitan Museum of Art*)

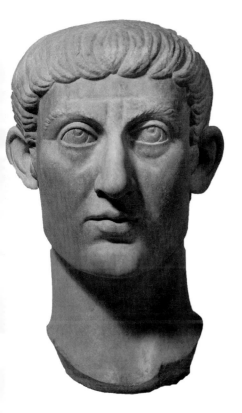

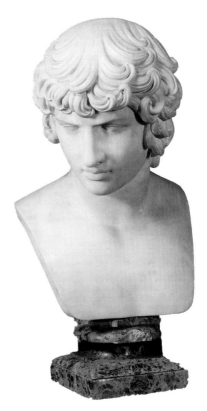

22. Constantine the Great, whose wife and son died in mysterious circumstances. (*Metropolitan Museum of Art*)

23. Bust in white marble of Antinous favourite of the Emperor Hadrian, worshipped in guise of Dionysius but here represented as a young man. (*Wellcome Collection. Attribution 4.0 International (CC BY 4.0)*)

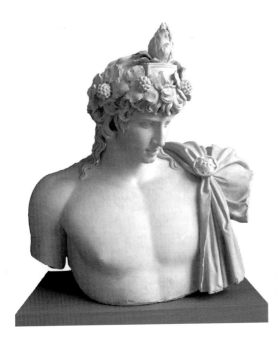

24. Braschi Antinous as Dionysos, plaster cast. (*Museum of Classical Archaeology, Cambridge no.470. (Original: Rome, Vatican Museums, Sala Rotunda, inv.540)*)

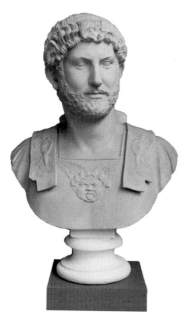

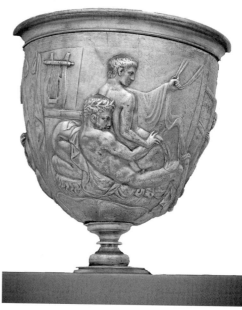

25. Portrait bust of Hadrian, plaster cast. (*Museum of Classical Archaeology, Cambridge no.531. (Original: Rome, Vatican Museum inv.1230, formerly Chiaramonti 392)*))

26. Image from the famous Warren Cup, now in the British Museum. (*Permission for use granted by the trustees of the British Museum*)

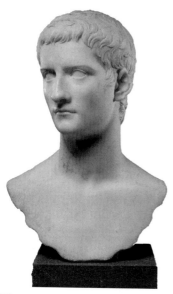

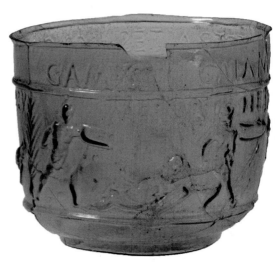

27. The enterprising Caligula, who set up a brothel in the palace. (*Metropolitan Museum of Art*)

28. Gladiator Merchandise in the shape of a glass cup. (*Metropolitan Museum of Art*)

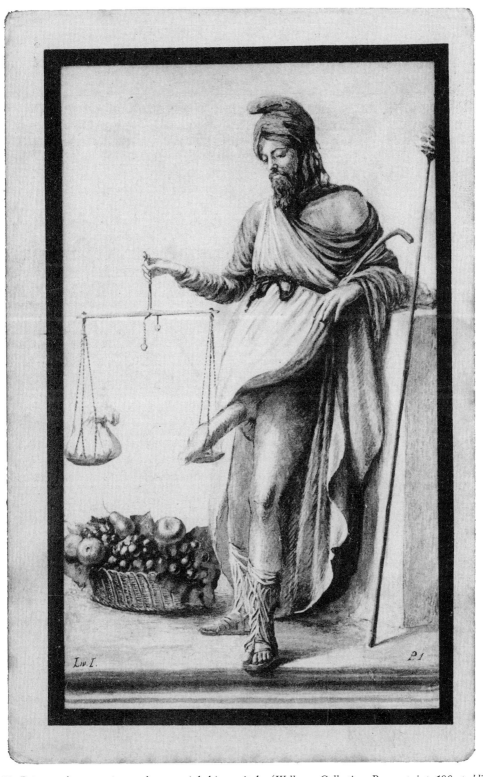

29. Priapus: A man using scales to weigh his genitals. (*Wellcome Collection. Process print, 190-.public domain*)

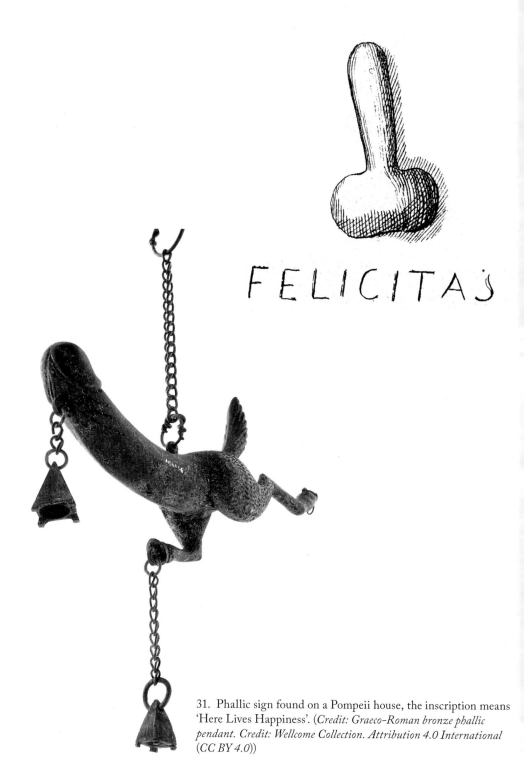

30. A very jangly hanging phallus from Pompeii. (*Credit: Wellcome Collection. Attribution 4.0 International (CC BY 4.0)*)

HIC · HABITAT

FELICITAS

31. Phallic sign found on a Pompeii house, the inscription means 'Here Lives Happiness'. (*Credit: Graeco-Roman bronze phallic pendant. Credit: Wellcome Collection. Attribution 4.0 International (CC BY 4.0)*)

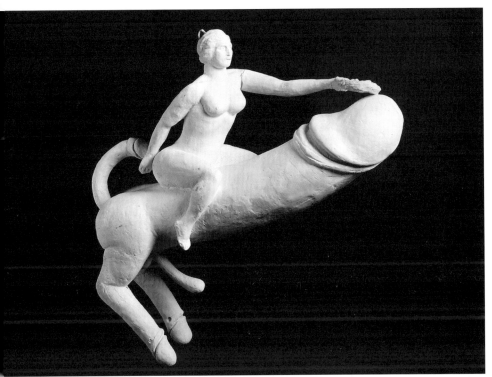

2. Plaster copy of an original phallus design (*Wellcome Collection. Attribution 4.0 International CC BY 4.0*))

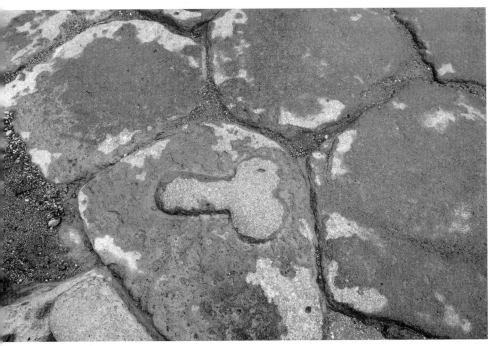

33. One of the many pavement penises in Pompeii, are they directing patrons to the nearest brothel? (*Seamer/Shutterstock*)

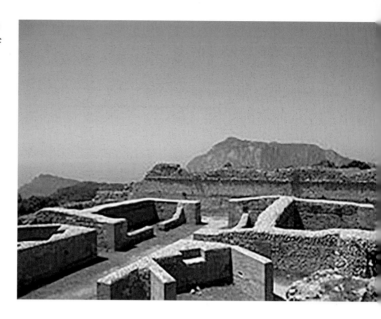

34. Villa Jovis on the island of Capri, where allegedly Tiberius got up to all kinds of depravity. (*Wikicoms*)

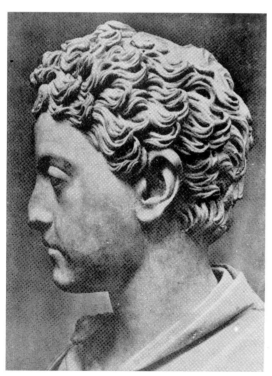

35. A young and innocent looking Commodus. (*Wellcome Collection. Attribution 4.0 International (CC BY 4.0)*)

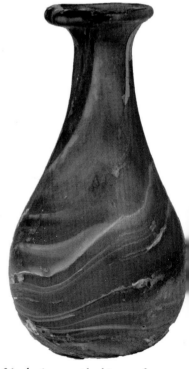

36. An innocent looking perfume bottle responsible for the decaying morals of Rome, mid 1st century CE. (*Metropolitan Museum of Art*)

Tiresias confirmed Jupiter's suspicion that women did indeed enjoy sex more and for answering honestly and revealing this secret he was struck blind by cross goddesses. A sympathetic Jupiter tried to soften this blow by bestowing the gift of prophecy on Tiresias. Not much of a consolation since being a prophet often involves telling people what they don't want to hear, which is what got him blinded in the first place.

This fear that women enjoy sex more than men undoubtedly colours the way they are represented in our sources. There is an ongoing motif of the insatiable woman, such as the Empress Messalina (who we will look at in more detail in a later chapter) who Cassius Dio describes as an 'adulteress and a harlot'. You'll be hard pressed to find a similar description in Cassius Dio of multiple adulterer Augustus or Julius Caesar.

Juvenal portrays her as utterly insatiable, servicing men as a prostitute all night long but still wanting more. Juvenal's satires are full of similarly insatiable women trying it on with actors, music teachers and even eunuchs. This fear that women enjoyed sex more is most likely behind a lot of the restrictions placed upon them: they could not be trusted with their own libidos and needed guarding.

Contrary to nature, law and customs – unacceptable sex

We've discussed above what was good and acceptable sex with the emphasis on mutual pleasure, let us now ask the question; what was unacceptable sex?

Handily, there is a book that answers this question for us and it's not a sex manual or an explicit poem as in Martial or Ovid, it is a book of dream interpretations. Artemidorus was a Greek living in the Roman Empire during the third century CE, and as a dream interpreter he collated the professional knowledge he had built up over his career travelling and interviewing people about their nocturnal mind wanderings.

The *Interpretation of Dreams* offers a real insight into the minds of ordinary people and the society they lived in. It's also kind of handy to look up your own dreams in, although be aware that Artemidorus does not mince words and will bluntly inform that your dream, pleasant as it may be, signifies your imminent execution as a criminal. Artemidorus has a whole chapter dedicated to sexual intercourse, which he subdivides into three sections:

- Intercourse which accords with nature, law and custom;
- Intercourse which is contrary to law;
- Intercourse which is contrary to nature.

Intercourse which accords with nature, law and custom includes sex with your wife, sex with prostitutes, sex with your own slaves, sex with a woman you know, and masturbation. In the second category, intercourse that is contrary to law, we find a multitude of unpleasantness around incest dreams, but the way Artemidorus categorises these dreams offer us quite an insight. In a section dedicated to dreams of having sex with your mother, Artemidorus says of these dreams, 'the outcomes they bring about vary with the various modes of contact and bodily positions adopted.'[6]

What follows is a comprehensive list of sexual positions on a sliding scale of awfulness/dire consequences for the dreamer. It's a distasteful chapter and I defy anyone to read it without wrinkling their nose in disgust, but what it offers us is unique: a comprehensive listing of what were considered, for the people of Artemidorus' time, acceptable and less acceptable sexual positions.

The very first position Artemidorus mentions is the straight-up missionary position, 'which some call the position according to nature.' Dreaming of having missionary position sex with your mother, should anyone wish to know, is very auspicious for artisans and labourers.

Next on the mother-shagging chart,[7] and moving into the more malign dream territory, is sex where your mother is offering her backside, as Artemidorus puts it, from which we shall assume he means anal sex. Then sex while standing up, followed by sex with the mother on her knees (doggy-style vaginal sex) or her stomach – the latter two of which signify complete destitution. Which isn't nearly as bad as dreaming of your mother being on top (the 'rider' position as Artemidorus calls it) which foretells your death.

Mixing up all of the above into a sexathon of variety particularly disgusts Artemidorus, who appears to be particularly wedded to the missionary position himself as the proper way to do it, and comments that, 'men also have a specific position, which is face to face and that they have invented the others when giving rein to abuse and lust.'[8] Which does make you wonder whether his own views on sex are colouring these interpretations.

At the very bottom of this depravity scale is to dream of being fellated by your mother: a dream that signifies the death of your children, the loss of all your assets, and, to cap it all off, a serious illness for yourself. Except that's not the worst outcome, as Artemidorus cheerfully adds, 'I know of someone who was castrated after having this dream.' Yikes! And we still have the 'contrary to nature' category to cover.

To summarise, sex dreams that are contrary to nature (according to Artemidorus) include dreams involving having sex/fellating yourself, penetrating another woman, sex with a god/goddess, necrophilia and bestiality. I don't think we want to delve any further into the latter of sections of this category: all you need to know is that terrible things will happen to you if you dream any of the above.

Artemidorus reinforces much of what we have already learnt, with one exception: all his interpretations in this section are aimed at men only. They offer quite an insight into the sexual freedoms allowed for men, having sex with prostitutes and slaves being deemed according to nature, law and custom, for example. In the section on sex with slaves, Artemidorus again makes the distinction between the penetrator and the penetrated: to dream of penetrating a slave (male or female) is auspicious, but to dream of being penetrated by your slave is inauspicious.

His list of sexual positions and adherence to the missionary position is fascinating, as is his own perplexation when two clients dream of performing cunnilingus and being fellated by their wives and nothing terrible happens to them. However, the matter is cleared up satisfactorily for Artemidorus when he learns the two men are frequent participants in these acts, 'So it was not surprising that nothing happened to them; they were simply seeing in their dreams what regularly gave them arousal,'[9] he concludes happily. This tale also shows that what Artemidorus considered contrary to nature and law was not shared by everyone else. Or alternatively, it was and breaking those laws and nature in a contrary manner added to the pleasure.

Chapter 9

Sexual Problems and Solutions

In the last chapter we looked at sexual intercourse itself, the good and bad, in this chapter we shall delve further into the sex lives of Romans by looking at some of the issues involved, such as contraception, abortion, impotence and fertility. But first up, what did the Romans understand about the differences between men and women?

Men and women

Roman doctor Galen was very clear on the differences between the sexes: 'female-kind is by nature colder than male-kind and for the most part stays at home.'[1] Women were also moist and porous, which explained their abundance of wetness whether it be menstrual blood, vaginal secretions or breast milk. In comparison men were dry. Being dry and warm is obviously more desirable than being wet and cold, but then being a man was wholly more desirable full stop.

Man was considered the norm, what a human being should be. Women were lesser, not just in strength and those cold, wet issues, but also because they were unfortunate enough to have the proper equipment to be a man but in the wrong place. Galen explains that a man's genitals are turned inward on a woman, the penis forming the vaginal passage and the scrotum the uterus. The testes in Galen's model become ovaries. In short, women were men gone wrong. Which might explain why, as we noted in an earlier chapter, Romans were so willing to believe that people could change sex. The parts were the same, after all, just differently located.

In a similar vein men and women were both thought to produce sperm, the relative strength or weakness of the combined sperm determined the nature of the child produced. Stronger sperm from the man produced a son, the weaker sperm from a woman would result in a daughter. The strength of the sperm depended on which part of the body it had been formed: strong parts of the body produced strong sperm. The resulting child would most resemble the parent whose sperm won out in that battle.

As you can see, medicine was very much used to enshrine the status quo regarding gender roles. However, there were some medical issues that affected only one gender or the other.

Men: trouble down below, impotence

There are few key requirements for successful sexual intercourse; two people, a location and an erection, the latter of which wasn't always so easily obtained.

> Yet I held her, all in vain, completely slack,
> lay there a limp reproach, a burden to the bed:
> though I really wanted it, and the girl wanted it too,
> I could get no more from my exhausted parts.[2]

So reveals the poet Ovid and he wasn't alone in suffering this problem. Horace also dedicates a poem to his erectile dysfunction. It cannot have been easy to suffer from impotence in ancient Rome, that aggressively male society where to be Roman was to be active, to penetrate. Those ubiquitous images of erect penises depicted everywhere for good luck must have really rubbed it in. As Artemidorus says, rather piling on the pressure, 'The whole principle of a family depends on the penis. It represents physical strength and manliness.'[3]

Just as women were expected to produce a family, so were men. As we saw earlier, men were just as included in the morality laws and encouragement of reproduction. Impotence, therefore, was a big deal. What methods did ancient Romans have for dealing with this complaint?

Horace and Ovid have different ideas as to what has caused their impotence. For the less than gallant Horace, it is all down to the unattractiveness of his lady friend, 'her damp cosmetics and her tinted make-up, dyed with crocodile dung won't stay on.'[4] Whereas Ovid suspects foul play in the guise of a curse or witchcraft (of which more later). A double case of it's not me, it's you.

Another impotence sufferer was the emperor Tiberius, who was said to have suffered from flagging passions in his seventies. These he tried to revive by collecting a huge library of erotic material and embarking on some seedy voyeurism. It does sound more fun than Pliny the Elder's suggestion of plunging an ass's penis seven times in hot oil and rubbing it on the limp part. I'm assuming that you let the ass's penis cool down first.

Pliny also notes, 'The right lobe of a vulture's lungs, attached to the body in the skin of a crane, acts powerfully as a stimulant upon males.'[5] If you can't find a vulture to dismember, an easier version is available in the shape of a cock's testicle (make sure it is the right-sided one) which should be attached to the body in the skin of a ram. There are no details on how a woman's libido is affected by her partner wanting to make love while accessorised by bird testicles.

Probably the least disturbing of Pliny's erection-boosting suggestions is to mix the yolks of six pigeon eggs with hog's lard, positively appetising compared with vulture lungs and ass penises!

Hysterical women

Medicine centres around fixing imbalances within the different constitutional makeup of the genders, and more particularly with women, dealing with their troublesome womb. The womb was thought to be a free travelling organ that could attach itself to other organs and cause illness.

One illness that affected only women was what was termed hysteria or hysterical suffocation. The key symptoms of hysteria were difficulty in breathing, talking and an assault on the senses. It might also include pains in the legs and groin and even seizures. The root cause was that troublesome womb not being in its proper place. It could be driven back there by use of foul odours: these could include burnt hair, or wool, even charred deer's horn which would be puffed up the vagina to repel that womb right back where it should be – and also presumably repel anyone in the room at the time. A doctor might also use a small pipe to further blow air up there.

Another way to shift the womb was by noise, a flute accompanied by a drum doesn't sound too bad, especially as it's recommended after a drink of wine (though admittedly wine doctored with other substances, in this case castoreum and bitumen). It might even be quite relaxing. Less so Xenophon's suggestion of beating metal plates together, after which the patient might well have a headache to add to her hysteria.

Gynaecologist Soranus is scathing about all of the above and issues what is probably the most sensible statement in all of ancient medicine on women's health matters: 'The uterus does not issue forth like a wild animal from the lair, delighted by fragrant odours and fleeing bad odours.'⁶ He even identifies other underlying reasons for hysteria, 'In most cases the disease is preceded by recurrent miscarriages, premature birth, long widowhood, retention of menses and the end of ordinary childbearing.'⁷ This very telling statement hints that hysteria was less of a physical disease and more related to mental health. Soranus' key remedy is to lie the patient down in a warm room to rest and sponge her face a little, which is infinitely preferable to having charred wool smoked up your vagina while someone bangs a plate right next to your ear.

Contraception

Contraception is split between preventing conception prior to sex and preventing it post sex. On the pre-sex side rubbing olive oil around the entry point is recommended, which presumably would work quite nicely as a lubricant as well. Certainly better than honey, which is another suggestion.

White lead, as well as rotting your face away, is given the opportunity to rot away other parts, too, when mixed with balsam oil and rubbed around the vulva. Other disgusting-sounding concoctions said to be effective (if you dare) include boiled mule testicles mixed with the juice of the willow tree and vulture dung. Although the success rate of the latter might well be down to the male refusing to have sex with someone whose lady parts are covered in bird poo.

Wool pessaries pop up (literally) as a suggestion. You have a choice here as to what you soak the wool in; honey or olive oil don't sound too bad, whereas crocodile dung certainly does.

On the entirely bizarre side, and if the repeated use of animal poo wasn't strange enough for you, apparently some women were wearing part of a lioness's womb in an ivory tube. Or, look away now if you're squeamish, cutting open the head of a particular spider, removing the two tiny worms found in there and tying these worms to themselves. One would hope these worms were tied somewhere discreetly, as they'd be somewhat of a passion killer otherwise. Pliny the Elder tells us that aconite rubbed on a girl's vulva will cause death sometime later, which is a form of contraception, I guess.

On the post-coital side, it's all about expelling the sperm. Soranus has a foolproof way of killing both conception and the mood, by requiring the woman to get up post climax, squat down, sneeze, have a good wipe around and then drink something cold. It's a very special man who sticks around for the final gulp of that ice-cold cordial.

For men, juniper juice is applied to the penis prior to intercourse. Although, given that Pliny also recommends it for dandruff and a nasty infection of the eyelashes, you might want to think about that one carefully.

Abortion

Childbirth was extremely dangerous for women in the ancient world as there was little in the way of interventions available if something went wrong with the birth. Grave inscriptions show an increase in female mortality between the ages of fifteen and twenty-nine years, the key childbearing years. Understandably, some women wanted to limit the number of children they had, and if contraception failed then the other option was abortion.

The Hippocratic Oath is the foundation of medicine, taken by newly trained doctors, it held them to a set of ethical standards of practice, and much of what was sworn all those centuries ago is still held to by the medical profession today. The line we can all remember is 'do no harm', but there is more to it than that: ethical standards such as patient confidentiality, 'whatever I see and hear, professionally and privately, which ought not to be divulged, I will keep secret and tell no one'; and acting appropriately in a position of trust, 'I will not abuse my position to indulge in sexual contact with the bodies of women or men.'

Also included is the line, 'Neither will I give a woman means to procure an abortion.' This would lead us to assume that antiquity held strong views on abortion, but later in the Hippocratic writings we find a doctor encouraging a pregnant prostitute to jump up and down to expel the foetus.[8] This contradiction troubles our doctor Soranus, who explains that two camps had formed, one that took the line in the oath as absolute and the other that maintained that abortion was allowed for solid medical reasons (though the example given of the prostitute is lacking in any medical validity).

Soranus nonetheless gives us a series of methods of abortion after conception, such as vigorous exercise, laxatives, travelling on a horse, rubbing oil into the body, particularly around the pubic area, bathing daily in sweet water after drinking some wine and living off what Soranus describes as 'pungent' food.

If none of these are successful then Soranus suggests more stringent measures: the sweet water bath is replaced by one of linseed, fenugreek, mallow and wormwood. The poultices get more hardcore: one is made of ox bile and absinthe, which boggles the mind. The patient is advised to prepare for these treatments by having long baths, abstaining from wine, not eating much and to use vaginal softening suppositories made up of wallflower, cardamom, brimstone, absinthum, myrrh and water, as well as succumbing to being bled. Soranus gives a less favourable write-up to amulets and mule uteruses, which he dismisses as quack medicine.

Evidently Romans knew how to perform a surgical abortion, and the Christian writer Tertullian writes of an instrument shaped like a hook used to remove a dead foetus from the womb. He also makes mention of copper needles used as an abortive tool, commenting that it is a furtive robbery of life.[9] There is not the discourse on abortion in ancient Rome that there is in the modern world, but there were Romans who very much did not approve, like Tertullian. Ovid is also critical of abortion, 'Whoever first taught the destruction of a tender foetus, deserved to die by her own warlike methods,'[10] he says after his mistress, Corinna, aborts a child.

Ovid also suspects that abortions are procured so that the woman may keep her figure. Juvenal, unsurprisingly, also harbours suspicions about abortions, speculating that they are a way of women ridding themselves of the product of their adultery. 'Why submit your womb to probing instruments, or give lethal poison to what is not yet born?' Ovid questions, and comments that often a girl who induces an abortion loses her own life as well. It was certainly not a safe procedure; it was inherent with risks. The daughter of the Emperor Titus, Julia Flavia, was said to have died after having an abortion.[11]

There were some laws passed on abortion. These are not about preventing the act but rather to punish those who sold dangerous potions that killed both child and mother. On the subject of abortion, we must remember that Rome was a society where newborn infants were routinely exposed: there was no concept of a right to life for either children or foetuses.

Fertility

We've discussed how to prevent and how to end unwanted pregnancies, but what if you cannot get pregnant in the first place? As we have discussed previously, the expected role of women in Roman society was to produce children; to not produce children was to fail in their duties. Infertility was a ground used for divorce. The Emperor Nero, for example, divorced his first wife, Octavia, for being barren and you'll remember Turia from a previous chapter who offered to step aside for her husband to marry another due to her barrenness. Alongside which we have those Augustan morality laws dishing out benefits for those who produced three children. There must have been considerable pressure placed on women, not least because any problems in conceiving were thought to be all her fault.

Doctors had a checklist of what a fertile and an infertile woman looked like: those who are mannish, sturdy, too thin or with freckles are likely to be infertile. But alternatively, if the woman is too flabby and very moist they are also likely to be infertile. Those who blush a lot are also likely to be infertile because that heat dries up the sperm. Fertile women, on the other hand, have good bowel movements and are cheerful.

Aside from her visual appearance, there were other ways to tell if a woman was fertile. Diocles suggests placing a pessary of resin, rue, garlic, nosesmart and coriander in her vagina: if she can taste these substances in her mouth she is fertile; if she cannot she is infertile. There is a similar experiment in the Hippocratic writings. Here, you wrap the woman in a cloak and burn incense (from a safe, non-inflammatory distance) beneath her: if the smell of the incense passes through her body to her nose and mouth she is not sterile.

Soranus neatly sums up all of the above, 'All this is wrong,' noting that fleshy women and thin women have conceived quite happily in his experience. His criteria for spotting the fertile woman is much simpler and doesn't involve anything being shoved up anyone, 'As a general rule one must look for a woman whose body as well as her uterus is in a normal state.'[12] He then ruins this simple and sensible statement on good maternal health being the key factor in fertility by entering into a laboured metaphor of seeds and land and crops, which we will pretend never happened.

That fertility was important to women is evident in the sheer number of dreams that Artemidorus records which foretell the birth of children. He also lists dreams as auspicious or inauspicious for the childless. That the childless have a special category of their own for dream interpretation is telling.

Fertility featured heavily in religion. During Lupercalia (in February) one of the rites involved half-naked youths armed with whips running round the city. Women would purposefully hold out their hands for whipping since it was said to cure infertility. The Temple of Diana at Nemi was a place of pilgrimage for both pregnant women hoping for a safe delivery and women hoping to fall pregnant. Numerous votive offerings have been found at the temple, including many votive wombs, which might well be a gift for the goddess to help with reproductive issues.

You could ask for divine help with your fertility, but was there anything medically you could do to aid conception? Timing was important: Soranus recognises that immediately after menstruation is an optimum time to get pregnant. He also suggests that you will more easily fall pregnant if you are firstly feeling well up for it, when you are not too full from dinner and particularly that you are not drunk.

Although Soranus' reasoning for the no-drinking rule before sex is not what you'd expect, it is nothing about optimum health but rather based on some notion that the mental state of a woman during conception affects the soul of the child. To back this up Soranus offers up cases of women who have seen monkeys during intercourse and gone on to have babies that resembled monkeys. Booze, so Soranus tells us, causes strange fantasies and makes people deranged – so for the sake of the child cut it out.

Sexually transmitted diseases

Given the license Roman men had to enjoy as much sex as they pleased (within cultural boundaries) both in and outside marriage, and the eyebrow-raising accounts of the sex lives of various emperors, not to mention the lack of protective contraceptive devices, we might assume that ancient Rome was a hotbed of venereal disease. Quite possibly, but identifying it proves problematic.

The ancient medical writers have a very different understanding of the human form and how the body works, they use different language to describe and explain functions. They also have a limited notion of how diseases, sexual or otherwise, are transmitted. All of which can make it difficult, even when presented with a thorough list of symptoms, to diagnose the patient's illness.

As a case in point, Soranus in his Gynacology has a chapter titled 'On the Flux of Semen'. Flowing seed in Greek is *gonos rhoos* (which is where we get the word gonorrhoea from). Soranus' chapter begins 'the flux of semen occurs not only in men but women too. It is a discharge of seed without desire or erection.'

Soranus, armed with the belief that both men and women produce sperm, thinks he is seeing the expulsion of sperm from the woman because of a lax uterus. To the modern reader what Soranus is seeing sounds more like a vaginal discharge, but we don't have enough details to back that up or to identify this discharge as a symptom of venereal disease. Besides which, Soranus is there present with the patient. Who are we to think we can diagnose better than he can over two thousand years later?

Soranus is not alone is noticing these symptoms, Celsus makes mention of a similar complaint, 'Here is also a complaint about the genitals, an excessive outflow of semen; which is produced without coition, without nocturnal apparitions, so that in course of time the man is consumed by wasting.'[13]

In the Hippocratic writings there is the case of Nicodemus who gains a fever because, we are explicitly told he had been overdoing it with both drinking and sex. Aside from his fever, he has a pain in his heart, his urine his thin and dark and he vomits up yellow matter. On the twentieth day of his symptoms the doctor records that his urine is thick and white: is that thick, white urine a discharge born of his sexual indulgence?

Another young man who had been indulging in too much sexual intercourse (as judged by the anonymous Greek doctor) presents with symptoms including fever, insomnia and a lack of thirst. By day twenty he was delirious and on the twenty-fourth day died. Is the doctor right in attributing his illness and death to all that sex he was having? Yes, but not in the way we would think of it.

The Romans had little idea how diseases, sexual or otherwise, spread. They had noticed that in swampy areas people were susceptible to a strange and often deadly fever, but they didn't make the link to a certain malaria-spreading insect. Rather, they explain illnesses on an imbalance of your humours, which can be influenced by the climate you live in and the direction of the wind.

It was agreed that sexual intercourse was good for the health, but too much was thought to sap the energy and could lead to illness or even death. That Galen terms this as a death from an excess of pleasure is telling, in the two examples above we saw that both young men had indulged in sex and drink. Galen adds to this list food and possessions, with a strong warning not to be excessive in all these activities because of the danger to your soul. Yes, we are back to our old friend *virtus* and the importance of character. This concentration on watching your appetites is almost akin to the modern notion of wellness – with body, character and spirit all interlinked.

But let us head back to gonorrhoea and other nasties of the genitals. Given the frank discourse in Roman society and the adherence to the public baths, where all who attended were naked, we might expect to find all manner of references to diseases of the genitals. True, Martial does write a poem making fun of a certain Catullus' (not that Catullus!) swollen testicles, and there is the case of Arria's husband who suffered an ulcer of the penis[14] alongside some moans about pains in that area, but there is surprisingly little. This doesn't mean there wasn't any, but rather that the difference in how the Romans understood disease means it is impossible to identify any sexually transmitted diseases with any confidence.

Chapter 10

Love Hurts: When Love goes Wrong

'Cynthia was the first, to my cost, to trap me with her eyes: I was untouched by love before then.' So says the poet Propertius of his mistress. Cynthia features frequently in his four books of poems, known as *The Elegies*. It's fair to say they had a tempestuous relationship. It's also fair to say that Propertius and Cynthia seem uniquely ill suited to each other. It was never going to be a smooth ride.

Propertius suffers; greatly. He spends a lot of time over four books of poetry telling us how much he is suffering. 'This madness has not left me for one whole year now, though I do attract divine hostility,' he complains. 'Let scorned lovers, after me, read my words with care, and benefit from knowing my ills,' he moans. 'This, the way of life I suffer, this is my fame,' he whines. 'Truly this is a silent, lonely place for grieving, and the breath of the West Wind owns the empty wood. Here I could speak my secret sorrows freely, if only these solitary cliffs could be trusted,'[1] he cries.

Really, he doesn't half go on about how miserable he is, and why is he miserable? It's all Cynthia's fault, she is serially unfaithful to the suffering poet and his poems are frequented with joyful nights, followed by deep despair when he discovers her latest infidelities.

I'm not entirely convinced that Propertius doesn't deserve this treatment as he whinges so very much. He is quite insufferable. This is best demonstrated by the line, 'You're my only home, my only parents, Cynthia: you, every moment of my happiness. If I am joyful or sad with the friends I meet, however I feel, I say: "Cynthia is the reason."'[2]

I think we all remain surprised that he manages to hold onto any friends at all. We get some sense of Cynthia herself via Propertius' whinging. He complains bitterly about her staying up late into the night rolling dice and drinking fine wine, he bitches about her singing obscene ditties, he's pained when she spends time in Baiae, the sin city by the sea. Basically, she appears to be having a lot of fun. Unlike Propertius, who is crying into his papyri and then going back for more.

At one point she tries to convince him that all these men kissing her are her relatives, so it's all alright. He is not fooled. She is like a moth to a light when it comes to gifts, flitting towards men who will buy her stuff. She messes with Propertius something rotten, after a joyous night (well as joyous as Propertius gets) a falling out inevitably follows.

She is very much the epitome of the 'treat them mean, keep them keen' mantra, and it works too. Propertius keeps going back for more, despite several hints that he is actually quite terrified of her.[3] I guess it provides good material for his particular branch of moaning in verse.

Also suffering for love is Tibullus. His beloved is Delia and she is unfortunately married, which complicates their liaison. However, Tibullus is quite enlightening on ways to conduct this kind of furtive affair. Delia has learnt to make excuses to her husband as to why she wishes to sleep alone, she can open a door quietly, and Tibullus, the gent, has given her herbs to sort out the bruises and teeth marks obtained during their sex sessions.

But if we want to talk suffering, heartbreak and poetry, there is one man who rises above all over poets in his pain, Gaius Valerius Catullus.

The suffering poet: Catullus

We met Catullus in our first chapter being gloriously abusive, but despite his potty mouth he was a nice, well brought-up boy from a wealthy equestrian family. Expected to follow a public career, Catullus moved to Rome to make the necessary connections and here he fell hopelessly, helplessly and touchingly in love with a woman he calls Lesbia.

That he loved her deeply is evident from the poetry he wrote for her, which talks of kisses that are never enough to sate him. These are beautiful, touching and tender poems, yet filled with the exhilaration of rushing, burning desire. There was a problem with Lesbia, though: she was married. Her name, her real name that is, was Clodia Metella, and she hailed from a distinguished but notorious family.

The Claudian family dated back to the time of Romulus and had produced a motley crew of ancestors, from the great to the good to the plainly batty. In the former category Suetonius tallies up twenty-eight consulships, five dictatorships, seven censors, six triumphs and two ovations for the family.

In the batty category we find Claudius Pulcher. In Rome it was standard before any important battle to consult the auspices to check that they were favourable for the impending fight. One such way of taking the auspices was by an observation of the sacred chickens: if they should eat some grain thrown on the ground it was a positive auspice, if they should refuse to eat it was a negative. Pulcher, frustrated by the chickens' refusal to provide him with a positive auspice, declared that if they would not eat then let them drink! And he tossed them into the sea, a scandalous act of impiety. The chickens won out, however, because Pulcher was defeated comprehensively in his sea battle and utterly humiliated. Never mess with the sacred chickens.

The Claudians would go onto to produce emperors Tiberius, Caligula, Claudius and Nero – a neat pick and mix of the best and worst of the Claudian traits. But in Clodia's time the most notorious of her relatives was her brother, Clodius Pulcher, described by Plutarch as 'a man of wanton violence, and full of all arrogance and boldness.'[4] He'd been causing trouble of one sort of another for years, including accusations of organising a mutiny in Syria and incest with his sister, Claudia, whom Plutarch is similarly unimpressed by, describing her as 'a licentious and base woman.'[5]

But his most recent exploit had caused an even bigger scandal: he'd been accused of putting on drag and gate-crashing the women-only festival of the Bona Dea. These sacred rites were being held at Julius Caesar's house and the rumour was that Clodius was having an affair with Caesar's wife, Pompeia, hence his unwelcome intrusion.[6] Alternatively, rites designated 'secret' and 'women only' are madly tantalising and it's not infeasible that it was a wild bet that Clodius was determined to win. Either way it was a gross sacrilege and Clodius ended up on trial.

During the trial a long line of witnesses were produced to testify against Clodius, including Cicero. It was at this trial that Clodius' ex-brother-in-law Lucullus brought witnesses to the court to swear that the defendant had committed incest with his former wife, though it was largely believed that Clodius was enjoying all three of his sisters. Catullus does make an illusion to this in one of his poems, 'Lesbius is pretty. How could one disagree? Lesbia would prefer him to you and all your family, Catullus.'[7]

Surprisingly, Clodius was acquitted, mostly because the jury had been heavily intimidated and bribed by the defendant's supporters. However,

Clodius had only got started on his career of troublemaking. He would spend the next few years persecuting Cicero in a variety of ways, including getting him exiled and in his absence demolishing his house. Also forming his own mob and using it to follow Pompey around, shouting rude things at him. By 53 BCE everyone had their own mob which they used to intimidate other mobs in order to influence the voting in elections.

Fame, notoriety, money and power all have an allure and perhaps this added to Clodia's attraction for Catullus. Clodia's husband, by comparison to her infamous brother, was the solid, respectable Quintus Caecilius Metellus Celer. He features in a few of Catullus' poems: in one he is referred to as a blockhead and a donkey. Cicero describes Metellus as 'not a human being. But mere sound and air, a howling wilderness.'[8] Which hardly improves the picture of him.

Whatever his personality flaws, Metellus was distinguished in service, having served as consul in 60 BCE and the usual positions required to get there. A husband was an impediment to their liaison, but there were other impediments too. Catullus was far from the only man Clodia was enjoying herself with, something that causes him immense pain. This pain pulsates through his poems, 'No woman can say she has been loved truly as much as Lesbia has been loved by me.'[9]

But also there is rage: 'I hate and I love,'[10] he famously says. He lashes out at both Clodia and those who have taken his place in her bed, accusing his beloved of wanking off men at crossroads and alleyways, of sleeping with whole taverns of men whom he threatens to orally rape, all two hundred of them. Also the subject of his rage is Marcus Caelius Rufus, a friend of Catullus' who cruelly betrays him, as he sees it. You can't help but sympathise with Catullus as his eyes are opened to his real position in Clodia's affections.

But as with Propertius and Cynthia, we only have Catullus' version of the relationship. Did Clodia ever promise Catullus anything more than an afternoon of enjoyable sex? It was highly unlikely that she would have turned over the distinguished, wealthy Metellus for Catullus, a young man on the very starting rung of his career. Did she ever even promise to be faithful to him?

She apparently once told him she would rather marry him than anyone else, not even the god Jupiter. But even in the middle of this passionate affair Catullus recognises it for the empty flattery it is. 'But what a woman says to her ardent lover one ought to write on the wind and the fast running water,'[11] he says dejectedly.

Catullus, for all his professions of devoted love, did not restrict himself to absolute fidelity. There is Ipsitilla, who the poet asks to stay home and prepare for 'nine consecutive fuckifications'.[12] There is also the young boy, referred to as Juventius, whose honeyed eyes Catullus could kiss 300,000 times and never be sated.

Catullus burns at Clodia's lack of faithfulness, but there's not a word about his own lack of fidelity to her, or even a recognition that sleeping with Ipsthillia and others counts as cheating. Of course, Clodia and Catullus are not married, but the lack of guilt or even questioning of his own sexual behaviour while raging against hers is quite pointed.

There is not, and there never could be, a happy ending to this story. Rome was a practical place, there wasn't much room for sentiment, for romance. Love poetry isn't about either, it's about pain and suffering and heartbreak, our 'whining to metre' again. Clodia and Catullus' friend Caelius' affair proved far more combustible, with Clodia accusing Caelius of poisoning in 56 BCE. There was a trial, the scandal of its day, and with Cicero representing Caelius, Clodia found her reputation shredded for all eternity.

Catullus died aged thirty, sometime around 54 BCE; Caelius perished during the civil wars sometime after 48 BCE, one of that generation of talented young men who died during a century of bloodshed. And Clodia? She gets a mention in a letter from Cicero in 44 BCE in passing but we know nothing else of her fate.

Chapter 11

Managing Affairs of the Heart: Religion and Magic

While Catullus has his pen to vent his hurt against the woman who has broken his heart and perhaps indulge in a bit of revenge by a public dismantling of Clodia's character, the ordinary Roman had other avenues for getting even.

The curse tablet was the go-to place to not only vent but get proper retribution against those who have wronged you. Given that Rome lacked anything resembling a working police force it is unsurprising that we find crime-related curses, such as this one, 'Docimedis has lost two gloves and asks that the thief responsible should lose their minds and eyes in the goddess' temple.'[1]

On the more trivial front (although clearly it was not trivial for some) the intense competition in chariot racing meant that their fans were prepared to go to extraordinary lengths to secure victory for their team. 'I call upon you, oh demon, whoever you are, to ask that from this hour, from this day, from this moment, you torture and kill the horses of the green and white factions and that you kill and crush completely the drivers Calrice, Felix, Primulus, and Romanus, and that you leave not a breath in their bodies.'[2]

Other curses are not so obvious, such as this curse against Tretia Maria, who has clearly done something dreadful for someone to invoke this against her, though we will never know what. 'I curse Tretia Maria and her life and mind and memory and liver and lungs mixed up together, and her words, thoughts and memory; thus may she be unable to speak what things are concealed, nor be able.'

Similarly, who knows what Tactia had done to deserve this fate, 'Tacita, hereby accursed, is labelled old like putrid gore.'[3]

Naturally, curses could also be invoked in the name of your love life to get even on a rival or to damn the ex who has broken your heart. Calling on help from the pantheon of gods or spirits was considered acceptable; less acceptable and considered more dangerous was magic.

Magic is surprisingly ingrained in Roman society. From astrologers and dream interpreters to potions and spells, magic was called upon by Romans large and small to manage their lives. Many of the rituals associated with magic were like those of the state religion, but the key difference between religion and magic was where it took place. Religion was performed in public in front of others, whether they be strangers at a festival or members of your own family. Magic was performed privately and in secret. For that reason, it often fell under the suspicion of the authorities and there were multiple instances of magicians and astrologers being kicked out of Rome *en masse* for causing trouble.[4]

Pliny the Elder was among those Romans who was cynical about the power of magic. He promises that he will never cease to expose the untruths of the magician, yet at the same time he dedicates a portion of his *Natural Histories* to charms, superstitions and incarnations.[5]

Magic was employed by individuals in their everyday life, whether it was a curse aimed at the git who'd stolen their cloak, or an amulet worn to protect them from bad luck. There are many surviving examples of spells, incantations and potions from the ancient world and perhaps, unsurprisingly, the majority are concerned with love. Magic offered a full range of services for whatever state your love life was in, from resolving acute unrequited love to getting revenge on your ex, or in the case of Ovid, causing his impotence:

> Has some Thessalian poison weakened my cursed body?
> Do charms and herbs hurt my poor self now,
> some witch transfixes my name in scarlet wax
> and sticks fine needles right into my liver?[6]

Which I think we can all agree is quite possible with Ovid. Perhaps some poor girl he tried chatting up at the Circus was after revenge.

At the milder end of the magic spectrum you might consult a dream interpreter on the meaning behind the nocturnal lustings of your mind. Artemidorus has a whole section on dreams about sexual intercourse. Dreaming of sex does not signify that you will be getting any shortly with the object of your affection, sadly. The penis, for example, symbolises both parents and children because of the seed it contains, so says Artemidorus. To dream of having it away with your willing wife is deemed to signify good fortune, while bad fortune is signified when the wife is unwilling.

To dream of having sex with someone you desire is deemed good practise for the real thing, says Artemidorus, 'Often a dream of this kind has helped the dreamer when coping with the mystery of woman, since the woman in such a dream also allows him to touch her secret parts.'[7]

To dream of held torches at night-time if you are young signifies 'love with pleasure and effect'. Walking upon the sea was another dream that was a portent of good things to come in your love life. However, to dream of running in a race for women foretold of a future working as a prostitute, and as we saw in an earlier chapter, anything involving intercourse with your mother indicated all manner of awfulness in your future life. These types of services were available to all and used by all, whatever their means.

The wealthy could afford to have an in-house soothsayer or astrologer, as the Emperor Tiberius did in the shape of Thrasyllus, whom he kept in his household to be available whenever the emperor needed a consultation. Although Tiberius soon soured on Thrasyllus and astrologers in general, banishing them from the city unless they renounced their profession. Perhaps Thrasyllus had been a little too honest about Tiberius' fortunes.

Although the utterances of soothsayers, astrologers and dream interpreters were very popular and a resource used by many, they were not free from criticism or cynicism. In a comic play by Plautus, a character's complaints about his wife include her hiring of magical specialists: 'Give me some money to make preserves; give me something to give on the Quinquatrus to the sorceress, to the woman who interprets the dreams, to the prophetess, and to the female diviner.'[8]

Similarly, Martial is fed up with paying a witch to exorcise the bad dreams his friend is having, 'Nausidianus, for our friendship's sake. Either dream of yourself or stay awake.'[9]

Unsurprisingly, arch cynic Juvenal has much to say about these types of people and the women – and it does appear to be primarily women – who hire them:

No astrologer lacking a criminal record possesses any talent,
[She] will consult him about the lingering
Death of her jaundiced mother (she's asked about yours already),
When she'll bury sister and uncles, and whether her lover will
Outlive her; what greater tidings could the gods bring her?[10]

Like in the Plautus play, Juvenal stresses how the women care more for their hired fortune tellers than their husbands. His chief complaint is that they distract women from their proper duties as they spend far too much money on what he sees as charlatans. There is a whiff of misogyny here alongside xenophobia, for the best in this class of professionals (and the most expensive) came from abroad.

Such cynical writings make astrology sound like a cheap con that silly women have been sucked in by. But there was a darker side to it, which is shown by astrologers being kicked out of Rome *en masse*, something that happened at least eight times between the years 139 BCE and 175 CE. What had they done to so offend the state?

It was astrology's predictive nature that made it dangerous, particularly when those predictions related to the emperor. In 20 CE Aemilia Lepida found herself on trial for numerous offences, one of which was asking an astrologer about the fortunes of the house of Caesar. This is where astrology becomes treason, the fear being that any prophecy relating to the emperor could incite the ambitious to make a claim for his role and cause public disorder.

The astrologers, dream interpreters and soothsayers of Rome were concerned with interpreting signs and offering advice on things deemed unlucky and so forth. But magic could also be used beyond interpretation and advice as a way of controlling the events of your life, such as securing you the love of the one you desire.

Ovid may have had those cool chat up lines and tricks to impress a lady, but not everyone is an elite poet with ample time to spare hanging out in public spaces trying to pull. Outside of festival days, and the multitude of days handily deemed unlucky for work, your ordinary Roman had a proper job that needed his attention. Thankfully, the Romans had an answer for the lovesick but time-poor individual: love potions.

Love potions pop up in several legal cases, which would suggest they were widely available and popular. Or at the very least there was a fear that they were widely available and popular enough to warrant legislation where they are interestingly thrown in with potions that induce an abortion: 'Persons who administer potions for the purpose of causing abortion, or love philtres, even if they do not do so maliciously, still, because the act affords a bad example, shall if of inferior rank, be sentenced to the mines; if of superior rank, they shall be relegated to an island, after having been deprived of their property. Where, however, the man or the woman loses his or her life in consequence of their act they shall undergo the extreme penalty.'[11]

Plenty of Romans believed in the power of the love potion. Rhetoric teacher Quintilian tested his students by setting them puzzling lawsuits. One such brain teaser was a pimp suing for loss of income after a young man gave one of his prostitutes a love potion.

Poet Propertius thought their potency could make even that paragon of historical virtue, Penelope, ditch her husband, Odysseus. Elsewhere, Propertius complains that his mistress has been unfaithful, 'Not by her morals, but by magic herbs.'[12]

Love potions ranged from the very basic, such as eating hare, which was believed to give the consumer a certain extra appeal for nine days, to the much more complicated. Here's the list of those magic herbs that Propertius complains about: 'He's drawn to her by omens, of swollen frogs and toads, and the bones of dried snakes she's fished out, and the feathers of screech owls found by fallen tombs, and a woollen fillet bound to a murdered man.'[13]

This potion starts off deceptively simple with some easy to obtain ingredients: 'Take pure olive oil and a beet plant and olive branches; and take seven leaves and grind them all together and pour them into the olive oil until they become like olive oil. And put it into a jar.'[14] So far so easy, but the next passage instructs that you should take your jar of potion up onto your roof, face the moon and say a particular set of words: 411 words to be precise and you must say them exactly right seven times for this love charm to work.

Another spell for binding a lover to you is inordinately lengthy and complicated. It begins with you making two wax figures of a man and a woman. These figures must be made in a particular stance with certain words inscribed on parts of their bodies. Next, you stick needles in specified places on the figures a set number of times saying particular phrases as you do so. After that you must write down all the words you have spoken on a lead tablet, 'And tie the lead leaf to the figures with thread from the loom after making 365 knots while saying as you have learned, "ABRASAX, hold her fast!" You place it, as the sun is setting, beside the grave of one who has died untimely or violently, placing beside it also the seasonal flowers.'[15]

And that's not the end? No, you also must write down and recite an incantation of over 1,000 words. Is it any wonder that Romans often outsourced their magical needs to the professionals?

Professional help came in the guise of witches and these are just as sinister as you would hope. As Tibullus describes here:

> Her spells split the ground, conjure ghosts from the tomb
> and summon dead bones from the glowing funeral pyre:
> now she holds the infernal crew with magic hissing.[16]

Tibullus' witch has him up in the atmospheric dead of night by torchlight as she conducts her spells, and she offers up quite an array of services. There is a spell that prevents the husband of his mistress, Delia, from discovering their liaison: 'He'll not be able to believe anyone about us, not even himself if he saw us in your soft bed.'[17] And one that Propertius certainly could have done with to save him a great deal of pain (and moaning), a spell to end Tibullus' love for Delia.

Horace has an even scarier witch in the shape of Canidia who uses human body parts in her spells, which she harvests in murderous fashion:

> So the lad, buried to his neck,
> His face showing like a swimmer's, chin touching
> The surface of the water,
> Might die staring at food, brought and taken away
> Two or three times each endless day:
> This so his marrow and liver, extracted, then
> Dried, might form a love potion.[18]

This suspicion of human body parts in magic pops up in Juvenal too: 'He'll dig into chicken breasts, the guts of a puppy, and now and then a male child; himself reporting what he has done.'[19]

This is horrible stuff, but then the use of magic was dark, and the Romans certainly saw it as such. Magic took away the free will of an individual by use of potions and spells and it could be darkly malevolent, as the following two spells demonstrate. This spell aims to break up the marriage of Apollonois and Allous: 'Let burning heat consume the sexual parts of Allous, her vulvas, her members until she leaves the household of Apollonios. Lay Allous low with fever, with sickness unceasing, starvation – Allous – and madness!'[20]

Other spells hint at a dark possessiveness. 'Do not allow her to have experience with another man, except me alone. Drag her by her hair, by her guts, until she does not stand aloof from me.'[21] This spell does not sound like a healthy interest in a girl, again it is very dark, nasty, malevolent. 'Do not allow her to eat, drink, obtain sleep, jest or laugh but make her leap out [...] and leave behind her father, mother brothers, sisters, until she comes to me [...] Burn her limbs, liver, female body, until she comes to me, loving me and not disobeying me.'[22]

The likes of Juvenal might have shrugged off the use of astrologers and other magic professionals as the whim of silly women, but there was real concern about the use of magic for malevolent purposes.

The mystery of the open window

In 24 CE a Roman official by the name of Plautius Silvanus did something entirely out of character and unexpected; he threw his wife out of a window.

Plautius was hauled before the Emperor Tiberius and appeared confused. He'd been asleep, he told the emperor, his wife must have committed suicide. He really didn't know what had happened. The emperor and others went to inspect the bedroom in question and there they found unmistakable signs of resistance, proving the falsehood of Plautius' claim that he knew nothing of this tragedy. With an ugly prosecution hanging over him, the now widower Plautius discreetly opened his veins with a knife to save further scandal.

The confused nature of Plautius' testimony clearly caused a great deal of speculative gossip for shortly after his suicide, Plautius' first wife, Numantina, was put on trial. The charge was driving her former husband insane by use of incantations and potions.

Numantina was acquitted of these charges and walked free, but the case shows how widespread the belief of magic was and how it could be referenced to explain the inexplicable. The Lex Cornelia was very clear on where the Roman state stood on the use of magic:

> Persons who celebrate or cause to be celebrated impious or noctural rites so as to enchant, bewitch or bind anyone, shall be crucified or thrown to wild beasts [...] Anyone who sacrifices a man, or attempts to obtain auspices by means of his blood, or pollutes a shrine or a temple, shall be thrown to wild beasts, or, if he is of superior rank, shall be punished with death [...] It has been decided that persons who are addicted to the art of magic shall suffer extreme punishment; that is to say, they shall be thrown to wild beasts or crucified.[23]

Magicians themselves faced being burned alive.

The magician on trial: Apuleius

When the writer Apuleius suddenly wed a widow many years older than himself it seemed inexplicable to the people around the happy couple. This marriage of opposites no doubt attracted a great deal of gossip, and then speculation, because Apuleius' bride was not only a lot older than him, she was also a lot richer. Questions were raised: so many in fact that Apuleius found himself on trial for having used black magic to secure Pudentilla's love.

We are lucky in that we have the full transcript of Apuleius' robust defence as this gives us quite an insight into what type of magic was performed in ancient Rome. Also, Apuleius' clear fury at such ridiculousness being slung at him is very entertaining, 'I think this is a sufficient refutation of the accusations concerning my hair which they hurl against me as though it were a capital charge.'[24]

Some of the accusations are laughable and Apuleius makes extremely short work of them, alongside his hair looking suspiciously magical we can add recommending a tooth powder to a friend, writing poetry which is a bit saucy (which Apuleius defends robustly with reference to Catullus), and owning a compact mirror which he looked into. His profession as a philosopher and the place of his birth, North Africa, are also used to suggest he is not entirely proper. A charge to which he responds, 'A man's birthplace is of no importance, it is his character that matters.' Hear, hear!

Apuleius is alleged to have kept magical items wrapped in a cloth in the house of his late stepson that he had constructed using secret processes and a seal for the purposes of the dark arts. It was said that he worshipped a mysterious object in his house and sought out a particular type of fish used in spells. And that he involved a boy in a dark magical process which made the boy fall to the ground. It turns out the boy in question is epileptic, so it hardly needed a spell to make him fall to the ground.

All these claims, which Apuleius gave short shift to for their ludicrousness, are to build up a picture of him as a dabbler in magic before the main accusation regarding his marriage. Reading Apuleius' defence, it's clear that the prosecution hasn't got much in the way of evidence to prove Pudentilla has been married against her will by use of magic. They read out a letter of hers that includes the line, 'Apuleius is a magician and has bewitched me to love him! Come to me, then, while I am still in my senses.'

This sounds a pretty damning accusation from the lady's own pen, until Apuleius reads out the entirety of the letter and the context changes the meaning entirely. In a nutshell Pudentilla's sons are put out by their mother having a sex life and remarrying, and another individual, who has brought the case against Apuleius, had run up huge debts on the expectation of marrying her. As Apuleius cries, 'You cannot even invent charges that will have some show of plausibility!'

If we substitute 'bewitched' for 'in her right mind', we find a very modern story of family dynamics, feuds and inheritances. Apuleius was acquitted of all charges.

Magic was a dangerous business to be involved in. But there were more acceptable, state sponsored ways to improve your love life, in the shape of religion.

Love gods

The gods were the go-to fix for the everyday problems that ordinary Romans faced. There are deities for pretty much every eventuality you could find yourself in, be it a fever, an arduous journey or a loaf of bread you've put in the oven and are hoping will turn out all soft and tasty.

Matters of the heart and sexual intercourse were no exception, and there were gods aplenty to aid in your love life.

Chief among them was the goddess of love, Venus. Venus Verticordia (meaning Venus the changer of hearts) was honoured in the Veneralia festival that took place on 1 April each year alongside Fortuna Virilis, which translates straightforwardly as virile fortune. Whereas Venus the changer of hearts was associated with domestic harmony and a happy marriage, Fortuna Virilis was linked to the sexual fortune of women. It makes sense to link the two aspects of life together, for who doesn't want a blissful married life with lots of great sex?

However, the two deities seemed to have been split in worship for the festival. Fortuna Virilis was honoured in a ceremony at the baths where women stripped off and bathed together. Added to this ritual were incense, poppies, milk and honey. The affair was strictly women only and it appears that these women were the lowly born and/or prostitutes. The respectable women, although they no doubt bathed in the sexual fortune achieved by the ritual, concentrated their efforts on worshipping Venus, changer of hearts.

The Vinalia, which took place later in April, was a festival dedicated to Venus that was specifically for prostitutes. They gathered outside the Colline gates of Rome and made offerings to the goddess, 'pray for beauty and men's favour, Pray to be charming, and blessed with witty words,'[25] says Ovid.

These two festivals highlight how Venus was not just about love but very much about the consummation of that love.

Another god associated with love was the son of Venus, Cupid. Cupid, armed with his bow and arrow, was less about marital love and all about lust and its ability to unhinge the sanest of people. Cupid had a less well-known brother, Anteros, who was the god of requited love. But that's not all. As noted earlier, there is a god for every eventuality in Greek and Roman religion, so alongside Venus, Cupid and Anteros we have Himerus, who personified desire without requited love. Presumably offerings were made to Himerus to free them from their terrible emotional state, possibly a god who would have been of use to our long-suffering love poets.

Ovid, when writing his *Art of Love*, was clearly channelling Hedylogus, who was the god of sweet talk and flattery. A bit more Barry White was Suadela, the goddess of romance and seduction, who can be neatly followed by Voluptas, the goddess of sensual pleasures, and then onwards to Pertunda, the personification of sexual penetration. And finally Pan and Priapus who are both linked to fertility.

Although religion was considered a better, safer, more acceptable avenue than magic, there were occasions when the state got involved. Much like astrologers and actors, people of certain religious beliefs could find themselves expelled from Rome. This happened repeatedly to Jews but also to members of the Isis cult, which was not so well integrated into state religion as the cult of the Great Mother, and was, on occasion, considered dangerously foreign. However, in the year 186 BCE a momentous scandal worthy of a *Daily Mail* moral panic arose over one particular cult.

Cult of license

'Whatever I say, you may be certain that it does not come up to the enormity and horror of the thing.'[26] So announced the elected consul of Rome, which I think we can all agree is one hell of a teaser statement. What was this horror to which he referred?

'Some of you fancy that it is a particular form of worship; others think that it is some permissible kind of sport and dalliance; its real nature is understood by few.' This particular form of worship to which he refers is the Bacchanalia. The Bacchanalia had come over from Greece to Italy sometime in the third century BCE. It was a mystery cult, which is to say that participation in the ceremony was limited to initiates into the cult who were all sworn to never reveal the details of the rituals. It all sounds terrifically exciting until you realise those rituals were most likely just offerings or sacrifices with prayers, probably a bit of singing and dancing, and probably some sort of sacred object to be venerated. I say 'probably' because the initiates were really very good at keeping their vow of silence and mystery cults remain happily mysterious to this day.

The Bacchanalia ceremony also involved singing and dancing, and, as you would expect given Bacchus is the god of wine, a fair amount of drinking. The idea was to let your hair down in honour of the god. Such ceremonies had existed in Greece for many centuries with never a scandal, but this was Rome, and as you should know by this point in the book, Rome was very concerned with public morals. A secret ceremony, you say? Taking place at night? With drinking? With men and women both present? You can see where this is going.

The account of the scandal comes down to us from Livy, who you will recall had the stated purpose in his history of documenting the moral decline of Rome, which I would argue hardly makes him an unbiased recorder of events. So what was going on under the guise of religious devotion? Livy tells us, 'When they were heated with wine and the nightly commingling of men and women, those of tender age with their seniors, had extinguished all sense of modesty, debaucheries of every kind commenced; each had pleasures at hand to satisfy the lust he was most prone to.'[27]

This is somewhat believable; people drink a bit too much, stuff happens, but then it all gets a bit fantastical. The whistleblower, Hispala Fecenia, describes nocturnal orgies where initiates were forced to defile others or submit to being defiled, with music being played loudly to disguise the screams of the violated. If anyone refused to participate, they faced being sacrificed or being tied to what Livy calls a machine which hurried them away to caves.

Men had sex with men, and in a frenzied madness shrieked out prophecies. Women dressed as Bacchae, with dishevelled hair, ran down to the river holding lit torches, plunging the torches in the water repeatedly, then holding them aloft to show that the flames still burned.

These accusations all come solely from Hispala, who falls to her knees in dramatic fashion after giving her evidence. Her tale is lapped up by the Roman officials who believe every word of it and they vow to crack down on this obscene cult. To gather more evidence the Senate offered a reward for anyone who brought a guilty person before them, or if they couldn't locate the guilty person to give the authorities their name instead. As you'd expect, this turns one woman's dubious testimony into a full-scale witch-hunt. The justification for this seems to be that, although there is not yet any threat to the state from this cult, there might be in future. 'So far, their impious association confines itself to individual crimes; it has not yet strength enough to destroy the commonwealth. But the evil is creeping stealthily on, and growing day by day; it is already too great to limit its action to individual citizens; it looks to be supreme in the State.'

Some 7,000 people found themselves on trial. There would have been more but many who found themselves denounced committed suicide rather than face prosecution, while others fled the city. Initiates who had not partaken in any of the alleged criminal activities, which included forging and murder, were imprisoned. The others were all executed, or in the case of women, handed over to their families for a private execution. Livy tells us that the numbers executed greatly exceeded those who were imprisoned: paranoia had truly hit.

Having dealt with the participants, the Roman state then turned its attentions to the cult itself. Shrines were destroyed and an edict issued that forbade the celebration of any Bacchanalia within Italy. There was a caveat though; you could still hold a Bacchanalia but to do so you needed to apply for a permit from the Senate and there were restrictions on what could take place, basically no night-time frenzied murdering or orgy type activity.

The Bacchanalia scandal is interesting for many reasons. It shows how paranoid the Roman state is about people meeting together in large numbers (for the same reason you find the cookshops closed or guilds disbanded). It emphasises again these concerns over moral behaviour, such as men and women drinking together in secret at night. But also, it is a story about how a suspicion of sexual recklessness can snowball into a murderous conspiracy. Which might make us think about how other stories of sexual recklessness in Roman history are told. Was there a slender nugget of truth behind the most over-the-top accusations of sexual excess about emperors that snowballed into the eye-popping, barely believable tales of Suetonius? It is worth considering.

Chapter 12

Adultery

From the exploits of Catullus, Tibullus and Ovid you could easily believe that adultery was an acceptable pastime for any bored young aristocrat and horny housewife. However, from the time of Augustus onwards, adultery was an offence punishable by law, and those punishments could be extremely harsh.

What counted as adultery was dependent on your gender. A man could be charged with adultery only if he had intercourse with a freeborn married woman, whereas sex with a married ex-slave, slave, prostitute and non-married freeborn girl were all acceptable behaviours and did not count as adultery.

This double thinking on respectability is picked up on by the poet Horace, 'May I never have anything to do with other men's wives. But you have with prostitutes and actresses, and so your reputation suffers more than your wealth.'[1]

By comparison, adultery for a woman counted as sex with anyone who was not her husband. Female adulterers, if convicted, could expect to lose half of their dowry and a third of their property. They could not inherit or receive legacies. They were no longer allowed to wear the *stola*, the attire of a Roman matron which signalled to all your married respectability. To lose this and your citizenship was to be reduced to the status of a prostitute. The cuckolded husband was compelled by law to divorce his cheating wife. Women whose husbands had cheated on them had no such rules forced upon them. On top of all this the convicted adulteress faced banishment to an island.

These rules were not just aimed at the elite senatorial class, they applied to all classes and positions in Roman society. There was a practical reason for the introduction of the Augustan morality laws, a falling birth rate.

It is always difficult to estimate demography from 2,000 years away, although many scholars have worked very hard at it, but given the high rate of infant mortality (as many as half of all children would have died before reaching the age of ten) Roman women would have needed to produce five or six live children to maintain the population level.[2]

The fact that Augustus brought in laws to encourage childbearing strongly suggests that this was not happening. Ancient Roman women had access to contraception and abortion, neither of which was terribly sophisticated or effective, but it was there and was used without censure. There was, of course, another form of contraceptive that most likely kept the birth rate down: slavery. Wives could easily bat away sexual advances from them towards their female slaves.

The low birth rate wasn't just down to women though, as one of Augustus' other measures shows: 'Certain men were betrothing themselves to infant girls and thus enjoying the privileges granted to married men, but without rendering the service expected of them, he ordered that no betrothal should be valid if the man did not marry within two years of such betrothal.'[3]

On the less morally dubious side there was another reason why the population was not reproducing itself. The period preceding Augustus' moral reforms had been one of devastating civil wars that had raged, with brief respites, for twenty years. The senatorial class had lost many of its promising men to battle. If you flick through Cicero's letters and tot up the names of his correspondents who were dead within five years, you begin to get a picture of just how traumatic the civil wars had been, though not only for the elite, because for every general or tribune there were hundreds of ordinary legionaries fighting under them who were similarly killed in action. Rome was an empire that relied on its army for survival, and that army needed to be peopled.

As well as resetting the population after the civil wars, Augustus set about resetting the moral tone too. It's difficult to know if the late republican era was more sexually charged than others or whether it is just better documented in the shape of Cicero's letters.

The notoriety of the era is best demonstrated by Julius Caesar, who was such a philanderer as to earn the epithet 'every woman's man and every man's woman'. We will ignore the accusation of passive homosexuality that every Roman politician attracts and concentrate on the former, because Julius Caesar was quite the promiscuous tart.

He has the charming habit of having affairs left, right and centre with his friends' wives, including the wives of his political allies, Pompey and

Crassus. He had a long-standing affair with Servilia, mother of the man who would be chief amongst his assassins. Even when abroad for work he couldn't stop himself having it away with the King of Mauretania's wife, and, very famously, Cleopatra.

He moved the Egyptian beauty to Rome, along with the child they'd produced together, and set her up in a house near his, without thought towards what his wife, Calpurnia, and mistress, Servilia, might have thought about it. This was a man who had the audacity to divorce his second wife, Pompeia, because of an affair she probably didn't have, based on the notion that Caesar's wife must be above suspicion.

Of course, that is not how the Romans saw Julius Caesar: all that philandering was exactly what a Roman man should be doing. Having an affair with a foreign queen, producing an illegitimate child with her and then inviting her to all the posh parties in Rome to rub your wife's face in it was acceptable, whereas marrying said foreign queen would have been wholly shocking. Something that Antony probably should have known about, but clearly didn't.[4]

Elsewhere we find Cicero divorcing his wife of forty-odd years and marrying his ward, who was probably in her early teens and forty-five years his junior. There's a very odd affair between Cato the Younger and Hortensius, the latter asking to marry Cato's daughter. When Cato refused the match, Hortensius asked if he could marry Cato's wife, Marcia, instead. Astonishingly, Cato agrees and Marcia marries Hortensius. Later, when Hortensius dies, Marcia moved back in with Cato.

Then there was Sulla, who divorced one wife for barrenness, married again a few days later and spent most of his day drinking with harpists, who were apparently considered wanton types (it's all in the plucking fingers). And we mustn't forget professional rabble-rouser, Publius Clodius, who wriggled out of a sacrilege charge by a combination of bribery and sleeping with as many people as possible to win their support.

If the men were dodging their duty to produce little Romans by excessive amounts of short-lived political marriages and sowing their seeds instead with foreigners and actresses, the women were also enjoying some freedoms – possibly because their husbands were away drunkenly fondling harpists and plotting their next marriage.

Again, the image of the independent late-republican woman may entirely be down to the amount of literature and letters that survive from the time. This is one of the few eras where we get a heavy thud of information on women, thanks to gossipy old Cicero.

Chief among those classy, go-getting republican women is one we've met before, Catullus' Lesbia aka Clodia Metella. Aside from breaking sensitive young poet's hearts, she seems to be having a whale of a time: 'debauchery, love affairs, adulteries, trips to Baiae, beach parties, banquets, drinking bouts, singing, dance bands, pleasure-boats.'[5] It's framed as a criticism, but let's face it, who wouldn't like to go to Baiae for a beach party and banquet?

Cicero claims Clodia has brought a property on the River Tiber solely so she can check out the hunks swimming there and pick one to seduce. Which again, sounds kind of fun and certainly passes the time if you're a very rich lady with not much else to do.

Cicero continues his theme of Clodia's wantonness, 'who prostitutes herself to every man, who always openly has someone chosen to date, into whose gardens, homes, and beaches of Baiae the libidos of all men visit by her.' Yes, it's rhetoric, and Cicero does a similar hatchet job on Mark Antony, but it's quite unpleasant, and you cannot imagine anyone saying the same about arch-cheater Julius Caesar. Clodia is married but her lovers are young, single men. Julius Caesar, similarly married, has affairs with his friend's wives. The latter, to our modern minds, is arguably worse.

From Cicero's testimony we are presented with a Roman woman with the freedom to enjoy life however she pleases with whomever she pleases. Which is quite at odds with the traditional Roman view of women and women's role in society. The Augustan legislation set out to reinforce these traditional roles: women were rewarded for having children, men were rewarded for getting married. There was to be an end to debauchery on Baiae beaches and marriage hopping. Welcome back to the golden age of Rome.

To promote this new tone, Augustus set himself and his family up as the example to follow. He demonstrated his commitment to matrimony by remaining married to his (third) wife, Livia, for over fifty years, despite their lack of children. He introduces his male relatives to public service by appointing them to positions serving the state at an (illegally) young age.[6] He also sends them to undertake military service with the legions: stepsons Tiberius and Drusus saw service in Germania, grandson Gaius Caesar was sent to Armenia, and great-nephew Germanicus was sent to help suppress a rebellion in Illyricum.

The emperor took a similar interest in managing the lives of his female relatives, 'In bringing up his daughter and his granddaughters he even had them taught spinning and weaving, and he forbade them to say or do anything except openly and such as might be recorded in the household diary.'[7] Suetonius records that when Augustus was at home he would only wear clothes produced by his women folk, and their contact with the outside world was also controlled by him.

Augustus' marriage with Livia was childless, but she had two sons, Tiberius and Drusus, from her first marriage and Augustus had a daughter, Julia, from his second marriage. It was Julia who was to suffer from both her father's views on acceptable roles for women and his dictatorial nature.

The rebel daughter

Julia was born in October 39 BCE on the very day her father divorced her mother, Sribonia, which was poor timing in the extreme. He'd done so in order to marry Livia, who was six months pregnant at the time with Drusus. As was standard in ancient Rome in cases of divorce, Julia went to live with her father and new stepmother, where she was brought up in the strict way described above.

When Julia was fourteen she was married for the first time to her cousin Marcellus, the son of the virtuous Octavia. It was to be a short-lived marriage, for Marcellus died unexpectedly just two years after they had wed. Two years later she was married off again to her father's closest friend and right-hand man, Marcus Agrippa.

Agrippa had played a pivotal role in Augustus' life ever since the heir to Julius Caesar had swept onto the political scene, aged only nineteen. Without Agrippa by his side it is arguable that Augustus might never have achieved the position he did. Agrippa's capabilities continued into Augustus' long reign and many of the successes of the era are down to him.[8] Being allocated the boss' daughter as a wife was a public statement of the high esteem in which Augustus held him, not least because Agrippa was plebeian by birth, which would usually have excluded him from consideration from such a marriage. It also designated him as Augustus' chosen successor.

When Julia and Agrippa married in 21 BCE she was eighteen and he was in his early forties. In nine years of marriage Julia had five children, a quite exhausting amount of childbirth. Her final child was named Posthumous, having been born after the death of his father in 12 BCE.

We can speculate how odd it must have seemed to Julia to marry someone she had known as her father's friend since childhood. But that oddity is overshadowed by who her father designated as her third husband, his stepson, Tiberius. Just to ramp up the incestuous nature of this union, Tiberius at the time was married to Agrippa's daughter, Vipsania. Julia was thus both his stepsister and his mother in law.

Leaving aside the dubious family connections, Tiberius might not have been too bad a choice as a husband for Julia: they were of a similar age, with only three years between them, in contrast to her marriage to the much older Agrippa. Under Augustus' enforced direction Tiberius had held a series of public positions with honour and had been a very successful commander in Germania. They had grown up together, so this was no arranged marriage of strangers. It was a huge honour for Tiberius, and, as with Agrippa, it was a public declaration of Tiberius' importance in the imperial dynasty Augustus had created.

They might have had a lot going for them as husband and wife had it not been for two crucial impediments: neither of them wanted to marry each other, and they were utterly incompatible in character and personality.

Tiberius' objection to the marriage was straightforward, he was deeply in love with his wife, Vipsania, and did not want to divorce her. Julia was not keen either. But what Augustus wanted, Augustus got, and so they were married.

The happy couple settled down into the type of monogamous relationship that Augustus fully approved of. When Tiberius got a little mournful about his former wife and followed her round the market with tears in his eyes, steps were taken to ensure that did not happen again. Tiberius was sent off to the provinces to bully the troops and Julia went with him. They had a child together, but when the infant died the marriage combusted spectacularly.

Quite what the starting point for this disintegration was we don't know. What we do know is that Tiberius abruptly moved out and refused to live with Julia. She made repeated complaints to her father about her husband

and begged to be released from the marriage. Divorce was easy to obtain in ancient Rome. The fact that Tiberius and Julia did not divorce therefore suggests Augustus put his foot down. They were to stay married.

However, Tiberius did not move back in; effectively they were separated. Julia took to the separation with gusto, intent on enjoying herself. To read the sources regarding this era, both primary and secondary, is to be presented with Julia as a positive nymphomaniac.

Seneca describes her as 'accessible to scores of paramours' and of prostituting herself in the Forum. Cassius Dio has a similar story about her drunken reveals on the rostra speaking platform. Vellius Paterculus names her lovers: Iulus Antonius, the son of Mark Antony, Quintius Crispinus, Appius Claudius, Sempronius Gracchus, allegedly among many others.

These are brazen public acts and one can only conclude deliberately so. By selling favours on the rostra, the very same platform where her father had announced his new laws designed to bring back a lost era of moral decency, Julia was surely making a point, or she just really did not care anymore.

Tiberius was certainly fully aware of her behaviour, because in 6 BCE he makes a very surprising move. Despite having been consul the previous year and recently granted tribunician power, he abruptly resigns from all his public positions and retires to Rhodes as a private citizen. Augustus was not happy.

The ancient sources, despite a general hostility towards Tiberius, are very much sympathetic towards him regarding Julia. Poor Tiberius, forced to divorce the wife he loved and marry this woman he did not: a woman who humiliates him so much with her brazen infidelity that he gives away everything he has worked for all these years to escape the public embarrassment of being her husband.

But let us take a step back and consider Julia's side for a moment. She was pressured into marrying Tiberius only months after Agrippa had died and she had given birth to her final child. Tiberius' reluctance to marry her was clearly well known and then there's that sad story of him following Vipsania around, crying. That's quite a humiliation for Julia, everyone in Rome knowing that her husband did not want to be married to her.

Then there was Tiberius' personality. Pliny describes him as the most gloomy of men, and Suetonius has this description of him: 'He strode along with his neck stiff and bent forward, usually with a stern countenance and for the most part in silence, never or very rarely conversing with his companions.'[9]

Tiberius comes across in our sources as an introspective man. Taciturn and cryptic, he was hard to make out and people struggled to understand him. He was a heavy drinker and mean with money. In his youth he suffered from acne and as an adult he developed an unspecified skin condition that left him with weeping ulcers all other his body. He was hardly dream husband material, despite his social position.

Julia on the other hand, in a series of anecdotes collected by the historian Macrobius, comes across as rather witty. When her father questioned her as to why the previous day she had worn a low-cut dress but today was modestly (and properly, to his mind) dressed, she replied. 'Today I am dressed to meet my father's eyes, yesterday it was for my husband's.'[10]

After a friend suggested she model her behaviour more on her father's taste for simple things, she replied, 'He forgets that he is Caesar, but I remember I am Caesar's daughter.'[11]

It was Tiberius who issued the first humiliation by moving out and refusing to live with his wife. Throw in a heavily restricted childhood, three marriages, six children and thirty-odd years of her entire life being controlled by her father, and who could blame Julia for wanting a bit of fun and freedom.

If we ignore the orgies on the rostra, most likely invented, were Julia's affairs any worse than, say, her father, who committed multiple adulteries, and whose friends collected virgins for him to deflower? Or the promiscuous Julius Caesar?

Of course, we are talking fearsome double standards here. Julius Caesar earned a nudge and a wink for putting it about all over the place. When Julia's antics reached her father's ears, she was banished to the island of Pandateria, a tiny spot that measured only 1.75km sq. Her life was again controlled by her father; she was allowed no wine and her father vetted all her visitors. Her unhappy marriage to Tiberius was finally dissolved by Augustus.

As for Tiberius, he eventually returned to Augustus' side from Rhodes and succeeded him as emperor in 14 CE. One of his first actions was to take away his former wife's dowry, restrict her income and ban her from receiving any visitors in exile. She was even forbidden to leave her house. He had clearly not forgiven nor forgotten his marriage to Julia.

Scandalous imperial ladies

Julia wasn't the only imperial woman wilfully flouting the adultery laws. Her own daughter, also confusingly called Julia,[12] was banished for the exact same offence. Exiled to the island of Tremirus, she gave birth to a child which her grandfather Augustus ordered to be exposed. As the paterfamilias of the Julio Claudian family, he was well within his rights to do so, but one has to wonder what were Julia's feelings on the subject.

Livilla, the sister of Claudius, carried on an affair with the Praetorian Prefect Sejanus, despite being married to the Emperor Tiberius' son Drusus. Sejanus is one of history's arch villains, lowly born he served in the Praetorian Guard, recommending himself to Tiberius when he saved the emperor's life during a cave collapse. But Sejanus had far grander ambitions than being the favourite of an emperor: he wanted to be emperor.

To become emperor not only did Sejanus need Tiberius' favour, he also needed to get rid of all those pesky family members who stood in his way as more plausible successors. He did this by fitting them up one by one on treasonous charges: this was how Caligula lost his mother and his two brothers. What would improve his prospects further? An imperial marriage cementing him further to the emperor, and that was where Livilla stepped in.

That Livilla was already married, and to the emperor's son no less, was no impediment. In 23 CE Drusus died very suddenly and unexpectedly, but at that point unsuspiciously. The widow Livilla was now free to remarry. Sejanus presented his suit to Tiberius and Tiberius said no. Livilla was a member of the imperial family, Sejanus, despite a promotion to the equestrian rank, was an ordinary Roman: the class difference was too great for Tiberius to feel comfortable. For once, one of Sejanus' schemes had failed.

Tiberius rejecting Sejanus' marriage proposition is interesting, after all, we saw how Augustus let his similarly lowly born right-hand man Agrippa marry his daughter. Perhaps this is a sign that Tiberius was not quite as enamoured of Sejanus as he appeared, or that he was a terrible snob.

Six years later, in 31 CE, Sejanus' dastardly scheming against the imperial family was finally revealed to Tiberius. The emperor, now wise to everything that had gone on, moved quickly and decisively, and

Sejanus was executed. Every associate of Sejanus' was also executed, even the prefect's two young children. His daughter, being a virgin, was not eligible for execution, so the executioner raped her before strangling her to death. Tacitus tells us, heartbreakingly, that the little girl had no idea what she faced and kept repeating to the executioner that she hadn't been naughty.

It was Sejanus' scorned and now childless widow Apicata who told the emperor of how and why and how his son Drusus had died. Apicata pointed the finger firmly at Livilla. Livilla's sins were manifold: adultery, murder and sleeping with a social inferior. Her mother, Antonia – daughter of Mark Antony and Augustus' sister, Octavia – took her daughter's punishment into her own hands: Livilla was bricked up in a room in the palace and starved to death. The same method of execution that chastity-breaking Vestal Virgins faced.

Messalina: the wickedest woman in Rome

The most (in)famous imperial adulteress is undoubtedly Messalina. Her very name conjures up images of see-through dresses, naked, oily limbs and lots of sex happening all over the place in one huge orgy. A quick internet search of her name brings up all manner of certificate 18 DVDs. 'I thought it might be sexy, but it's just porn,' moans one unhappy viewer of such a film.

She is the main character of an opera from 1899 that was so beloved of Toulouse-Lautrec it features in one of his paintings. He wasn't the only painter to use her as a subject, Gustav Moreau, Hans Makart and Peder Severin Kroyer, amongst many others, used their skills to depict Rome's most notorious loose woman.

Messalina is also beloved of pulp fiction which, with typical advertising flair, declares her 'The Wickedest Woman in Rome! The Woman who led an empire into an era of dark depravity!' And my all-time favourite: 'She was beautiful, sadistic, tantalising and deadly from the top of her golden hair to the tips of her silver whip!'

So, let us ask the question, is Messalina's reputation as a wicked, depraved, frequently naked humping woman justified? You will be pleased to know that yes, it is.

Valeria Messalina was born sometime between 17 and 20 CE as a member of the imperial family, with all the complicated connections that the frequently intermarrying Julio Claudian Dynasty had built up. Her great-grandparents were Mark Antony and Octavia, Augustus' sister. They had two daughters, both named Antonia. The younger Antonia married the brother of Emperor Tiberius and produced Germanicus (father to Caligula), Claudius and Livilla (who she had bricked up in the palace and starved to death). The elder Antonia married Domitius Ahenobarbus and produced three children. Their son, also named Ahenobarbus, went on to father Nero, and their younger daughter, Domitia Lepida, was the mother of Messalina. Which makes Messalina very well connected to the emperors of Rome. She was the great-great niece of Augustus, a third cousin to Caligula, a second cousin to Claudius and a cousin of Nero.

There is also a connection to Emperor Tiberius, but it is far too complicated for me to work out. Tiberius' brother was married to Messalina's grandmother's sister, which would make her ... answers on a postcard please.

In 38 CE, aged around twenty, Messalina was married to her second cousin, Claudius, who was forty-seven years old at the time. Messalina was to be his third wife. Suetonius tells us that Claudius divorced his second wife, Aelia Paetina, for trivial reasons, and his first wife, Plautia Urgulanilla, because she was suspected of murder. Which you would think would be the starting point for a truly juicy anecdote, but, unforgivably, this is the only time Suetonius mentions it.

Messalina dutifully pops out an heir, in the shape of her son, Britannicus (so named after his father's conquest of Briton), and a daughter, Octavia, who will, like other imperial women, serve as a useful bridge to hold the sprawling family together by use of strategic marriage making.

She also embroils herself in some high-level palace intriguing in league with the palace freedmen. These are not always terribly sophisticated schemes. Appius Silanus met his end over a dream. The emperor's close freedman, Narcissus, had dreamt in vivid detail that Appius Silanus had meant Claudius harm. Alarmed, Narcissus ran off to inform the emperor. Midway through telling his tale, Messalina gasped, and, with a shaking voice, told Claudius that she'd had exactly the same dream about Silanus the previous night, and on other nights too. Yes, of course Narcissus and Messalina had cooked this scheme up together, but, unsophisticated as it was, it worked, and the hapless, entirely innocent Silanus was executed.

This is standard palace scheming. The Julio Claudian dynasty, the imperial household and the entire senatorial class are full of people scrabbling for prominence and who are prepared to do whatever is necessary to achieve this. The palace freedmen are both prominent and powerful in this era: Narcissus, Callistus and Pallas are implicitly trusted by the emperor and he relies almost entirely on their counsel, much to our source's disgust. There is also likely a layer of insecurity colouring Messalina's actions, because her husband had only become emperor due to a happy accident.

In the wake of Caligula's brutal assassination, the Praetorian Guard had stumbled across the deceased emperor's uncle, Claudius, hiding behind a curtain. As protectors of the emperor, the guards needed one to protect, otherwise they were all facing mass redundancy, and Claudius was a member of the imperial family, so why not? They picked him up and carried him off to make him emperor.

Messalina, and indeed Claudius, could not help but be aware that the palace was littered with relatives who might have a slightly better claim on the title. Not least Caligula's surviving sisters who could boast a direct descendance from Augustus via his only daughter, Julia. They both had husbands who perhaps looked more imperial than Messalina's husband; they didn't slobber from their mouth and were not possessed of a tic to the head. Regrettably, Romans considered the disabled distinctly lesser people. Claudius' own mother described him as a half formed monster, and you'll remember from an earlier chapter how the exterior of a Roman male was thought to reflect his interior worth.

Such belief most likely explains some of the targeted scheming at members of the imperial household themselves. A sister of Caligula, one of the many Julias that litter the imperial family, was banished and later executed due to some cooked-up allegations from the empress. Her motive in this case was that Julia was exceptionally beautiful and the emperor was fond of her. One of her failed schemes was an attempt to assassinate the young Nero. This failed, it was said, when the assassins were scared away by two snakes that darted out from under his pillow. Nero's mother, Agrippina, another one of Caligula's sisters, very wisely kept her head down during this period, but still was targeted and persecuted by Messalina. Enough of this political intrigue, where's all the sex? I hear you cry. Well ...

Remember Silanus? He was executed because of a fake dream. He earned his visit to the executioner because he would not give in to Messalina's lust. Another man who resisted the empress was Marcus Vinicius, husband to an imperial Julia, who was also killed for refusing to meet the empress's sexual demands.

Then we have the actor Mnester. He is vaguely famous for having been a lover to Caligula, and Messalina was most put out that he would not consent to being her lover, despite making copious promises to him and 'frightening him', as Cassius Dio tells us.

Frightening someone, one suspects, is not conducive to producing the necessary ardency in a man, and so it was with Mnester. However, Messalina was not one to give up and she finally got the actor into bed by getting her husband to tell him that he must obey the empress in all things. Of course, the clueless Claudius was unaware that heavy humping was the obeying his wife had in mind. This is apparently how she obtained quite a few of her lovers.

Messalina was undoubtedly beautiful, and given the practise she got, probably great in bed too, but the above neatly demonstrates the ethical dilemma facing many a prominent man: upset the empress by not sleeping with her and face death or upset the emperor by sleeping with her and face death.

There was, though, an alternative, as demonstrated by Sextus Traulus Montanus, an apparently handsome equestrian who Messalina sent for and then when he arrived took an instant dislike to him and sent him away. Quite why the empress so disliked him on sight is open to debate. A pungently offensive perfume? A distracting mole? Or perhaps he was just so good-looking that Messalina knew she couldn't compete.

However, copious affairs with whomever she wanted, whether they wanted to or not, began to get a bit samey, a bit too ordinary, for Messalina. She needed something more. Tacitus is characteristically mealy mouthed about this, talking about Messalina's boredom and her drifting into 'unfamiliar vices'. What were these unfamiliar vices? Thankfully, we have other accounts of the era that do not spare our blushes.

Cassius Dio reports that the empress compelled other women to commit adultery while their husbands looked on. Pliny the Elder tells us Messalina once competed against a famous prostitute for how many men they could sleep with in a single day: the empress won with a tally of twenty-five different men. Juvenal claims she set herself up as a prostitute with the nickname 'The Wolf Girl' in a local brothel, and was still unsated at the end of the day. These are the stories that have fed into hundreds of historically inaccurate porn movies.

We do have to question how true these tales are. While many of her lovers are named in our sources, the prostitution stories lack similar details. That Messalina put it about rather a lot is a given, but these stories feel like a progression on these details: 'Have you heard what that harlot empress is up to now?' Gossip, in other words. The prostitute competition and the brothel stories are probably an invention.

However, do not despair for there is one hugely shocking Messalina tale that likely has some truth to it. It is the most shocking of all the stories, and our sources can't quite believe it happened: Messalina got married.

Tacitus paints it as the act of a woman who has committed every possible outrage going and this is the only one left that can beat the previous ones. The most extreme, scandalous thing she could possibly do, because after winning a sex competition against a prostitute there isn't anywhere else you can go. Marriage is the only truly shocking thing left to her.[13]

The story of Messalina's wedding it almost farcical. It really does underline how ignorant Claudius was of his wife's activities, how much of a dupe he was and how the real power in the Imperial household had lain not with him but with his freedmen.

The intended groom was Gaius Silius, who Tacitus, always sparing on the compliments, describes as 'the best-looking young man in Rome'. So obviously Messalina had to give him a try. Unlike Sextus, there was nothing repellent about Silius, and soon she was infatuated with him. So much so that she forced him to divorce his wife. Silius wasn't keen, but he didn't really have much choice in the matter, so he did. Tacitus cynically comments, 'The affair was lucrative.'

With Silius' wife disposed of, he settled down to be a fully kept man. A kept man who was showered with gifts from the palace, including some of the palace furniture and a cohort of imperial slaves to wait on him while he lounged on his purple dining couch. It was a good life, which Silius might have enjoyed for a nice amount of time had he not married the empress.

The sources disagree as to whose idea the marriage was. Tacitus says it was Silius' idea and that Messalina had been initially unenthused until the outrageousness of it appealed to her. Cassius Dio is of the firm opinion that it was all Messalina's idea and that Silius was the reluctant one. Both stories could likely be true, based on the respective parties blaming each other in the aftermath of events.

If you are going to bigamously marry your famously attractive boyfriend it is wise to wait until your husband is out of the way, which they did: Claudius was away in Ostia. As it was autumn, Silius and Messalina settled on a grape-harvest theme for their wedding, incorporating elements of the god Bacchus. The bride, hair worn loose for the natural look, accessorised with a Bacchic wand. The groom wore an ivy wreath and calf-high sandals. The wedding entertainment put on for the guests included a chance to watch the wine presses at work and there were women dressed in animal skins pretending to be maenads. We can only be grateful that nobody thought to throw some satyrs into the mix.

The question hangs in the air: what were they thinking? I think it's clear that Messalina and Silius weren't thinking. It was all a bit of a wheeze: a nice party, lots of booze, lots of fun and a further chance for the empress to be outrageously outrageous! But this was a formal marriage ceremony and Silius had just married the empress while the emperor was away. It could easily be spun as less of a party and more of a coup.

She'd got away with it for so long: the sexual indiscretions, the multiple affairs, sleeping with whomever she wanted as often as she wanted. Everyone in Rome knew about it, except her husband, and the reason he didn't was because those all-powerful freedmen had kept the truth from him. That was about to change.

While enjoying her wedding party, Messalina was wholly ignorant of what she had done. The palace freedmen were enormously rich and powerful because the emperor allowed them to be. They benefited hugely from the current regime and didn't want a new emperor in the shape of Silius. Where was the benefit to them?

The all-powerful trio of Narcissus, Pallas and Callistus were palace old-timers who had survived the reigns of the three previous emperors. Callistus had certainly had a hand in the death of Caligula, Pallas had played an important role in the downfall of Sejanus and Narcissus had worked with Messalina to bump off all those men who wouldn't have sex with her. These were hard, clever and ruthless men. Messalina had badly miscalculated them and she was going to pay the price for that.

Claudius was told. If you're expecting apocalyptic rage and screams of vengeance, think again. Claudius' response is oddly touching and real. He was confused and very shocked. 'Am I still emperor?' he asked his advisors again and again as he tried to take in the enormity of what he'd been told. Not only was his wife a harlot, not only was he the last person to discover this, but she was right at that moment working to displace him with her younger model.

Having put their own lives on the line by delivering this bad news to the emperor, the trio pushed the emperor for action. They knew he was weak, they knew that Messalina could turn him to her side, and they knew that once she did, she would seek vengeance on them all. The emperor was not in a state for decisive action, he was in shock, veering between condemnation of his wife and misty-eyed reminiscences of their marriage and their two beautiful children. It was down to them to do the acting. Narcissus took charge, transferring the command of the palace guard over to himself for one day.

Meanwhile back in Rome rumours were reaching the newly married couple that the emperor was in full knowledge of their antics. This rather ruined the party and the guests scattered, heading home for safety. The groom decided to head to the Forum, apparently to pretend he had been doing business there the whole time and knew nothing about this wedding malarkey. The bride hit upon the very thing that had terrified the freedmen, she would appeal to her husband directly.

Claudius was on his way back to Rome, travelling in the imperial carriage, when beside the road appeared Messalina. Shedding copious tears, she begged her husband to listen to her, the mother of their children, but a quick-thinking Narcissus yelled over her so Claudius couldn't hear her pitiful pleas.

Claudius was still vacillating, so once again Narcissus took charge, taking the emperor to Silius' house. Here, on full display, were the objects (and slaves) purloined from the palace, including some items that had belonged to Claudius' father. This roused his anger enough for Narcissus (again) to persuade him to make a short address to his loyal guards.

A bloody retribution ensued. Silius' pretence that he had been in the Forum the whole time and knew nothing quickly crumbled under the weight of imperial staff suddenly weighing in with details of Messalina's years of misdeeds. He was swiftly executed. Others followed: equestrians, senators, a commander of the watch, and a superintendent of a gladiator school, proving that Messalina really didn't have a type.

Not all connected with Messalina were bumped off, however. Sullius Caesoninus escaped execution because, we are told, his part in the parties was 'female'. By which we may assume he was the penetrated rather than the penetrator, or at least claimed he was. No Roman could believe that any Roman man could admit such shameful behaviour so Caesoninus got to enjoy his life, if not his reputation.

What of Messalina? She still hoped to talk her husband round and the emperor was dangerously softening. Before he could completely turn to forgiveness in stepped Narcissus again and ordered the execution that Claudius couldn't bear to. Messalina, finally realising her time was up, tried to stab herself before anyone else could. As she struggled with the dagger, lacking the courage to plunge it into herself, the guards broke down the door and did what she could not. When Claudius was informed he asked for more wine and went on with his dinner party.

As we've seen, Augustus' harsher penalties for adultery had little effect on moderating the behaviour of his own relatives, and within the general population it was clear that women were seeking out loopholes to get round the law. One loophole they'd discovered was to register as prostitutes. Suetonius views these women as purposefully giving up the rights and privileges of a Roman matron, debasing their status. This is evident by the wording of the law Tiberius introduced to close this loophole, which rates working as an actress as being on a par with prostitution. 'A woman who gratuitously acts as a bawd for the purpose of avoiding the penalty for adultery, or hires her services to appear in the theatre, can be accused and convicted of adultery under the Decree of the Senate.'[14]

Both Suetonius and Tacitus are clear these are notorious, immoral and shameful women. But it's worth considering whether they are simply making a practical decision. Being charged with adultery meant a Roman woman was stripped of her privileges and rank, and likely banished to somewhere not very nice. Clearly enough women thought it preferable to strip themselves of their rank and have sexual freedom with no banishment – otherwise it would not have been necessary to tighten up the law.

Tacitus names an elite woman, Vistilia, who registered as a prostitute and was exiled to Seriphos. Vistilia's husband is censured for not reporting his wife to the (moral) authorities. The reason, we can assume, being that he knew exactly what she was doing.

Perhaps the Lex Julia laws never could be effective, because they were firmly aimed at recreating an age that had probably never existed. No law could recreate this world, but it didn't stop emperors from trying.

Next up as the morality police was the emperor Domitian, who ruled from 81–95 CE. He set himself up in the Augustan model with an emphasis on building stuff that was practical and pretty, venerating the gods properly and sorting out public morals (again).

Of all the moral legislating that Domitian did (banning of castration and prostitution of freeborn boys) he went biggest on adultery, adding to the punitive measures issued against women who were found guilty. Under the Augustan legalisation, an adulterous woman could no longer wear the *stola*, a very public statement on a woman's moral behaviour, or lack thereof. Domitian added to this by forbidding them to ride in litters. All could see that a woman was shameful, and it probably cut down on the number of quickies taking place in passing transportation. Another law of his was to ban women convicted of adultery from receiving a legacy or an inheritance, which had been an important means for women to achieve some kind of independence.

Aside from this, Domitian also closed some of the further loopholes from the Augustan laws that had been exploited. Under the Augustan law husbands were forced to divorce their cheating wives, but there was evidence that they were then remarrying them. Domitian cracked down on this. Just like that moral reformer Augustus, Domitian was subject to cries of hypocrisy and double standards, as he was breaking the very laws he created.

The new moral hypocrite

Domitian was the younger son of Vespasian who had entered the race to become emperor in 69 CE, the Year of the Four Emperors. When Vespasian was declared emperor, he was happily hanging out in the warm climate of Syria. The eighteen-year-old Domitian, however, was in Rome and was thrust forward as the face of this new Flavian dynasty.

Vespasian made it to Rome to claim his laurel wreath around the end of 70 CE when he discovered his younger son had got married in his absence. The unexpected daughter-in-law, Domitia, had an impressive lineage, her father was the celebrated general Corbulo and her mother was a descendent of Augustus. This was useful currency in establishing a new ruling family whose own lineage was not nearly so impressive. True, Domitia had already been married when Domitian began courting her, but divorce was common and easy in ancient Rome and lacked any stigma. The divorce did not detract from Domitia's suitability as a bride.

Vespasian, however, was not pleased. Not only because Domitian had married without his permission as the paterfamilias, but also because he already had a bride in mind, his granddaughter and Domitian's niece, Julia. Julia was ten years Domitian's junior and the daughter of his elder brother, Titus, and a marriage between them would cement the Flavian bloodline. However, Domitian, we are told persistently, refused the match and stuck fast to his choice of Domitia.

The marriage between Domitian and Domitia did not run smoothly. There were rumours she'd enjoyed a liaison with her brother-in-law, Titus. Then in 81 CE, shortly after Domitian succeeded his brother as emperor, there occurs an almighty ruckus in their marital relations.

The sources disagree on exactly what happened, but they are in general agreement that Domitia was banished for adultery with the actor, Paris. Cassius Dio states that Domitian had to be talked down from executing his wife and that he murdered her lover, Paris, in the middle of the street. Which sounds a little unlikely, for surely he could have just dragged Paris to the palace for a more private death.

The suggestion lurking below the surface here is that Domitian had caught Domitia and Paris in flagrante. There was an archaic Roman law that permitted the murder of an adulterer and the adulteress wife if found in the act. There's little evidence it was ever enacted, and it was subject to frequent debate on the exact circumstances it could be used as a defence. But the point is made in this tale that only Paris is killed, not Domitia as the adulterous wife. Cassius Dio also claims that Domitian divorced Domitia, although he is the only one of our sources that says this.

Under his own laws Domitian should have divorced his wife. Domitia should have been stripped of her citizenship and reduced to the status of a prostitute, thus preventing any future marriage. She should have been socially damned for the rest of her life, but this is not what happens.

How long Domitia spent in exile is unknown. She disappears from the coinage for a short while, but what is known is that she came back. Our sources say Domitian was forced into recalling his wife due to pressure from the public, but this is likely an excuse. Domitian was altogether authoritarian and of a hard moral stance, and it's hard to believe he would bend to the will of the Roman populace. Let us assume he was the one who wanted Domitia back, for the entirely plausible reason that he missed her and loved her.

So here we have the great moral crusader breaking his own adultery laws multiple times. He either did not divorce his adulterous wife or remarried her, both of which he'd firmly prohibited. Domitia is not stripped of her status, and continues to ride in litters and wear the *stola*, again in breach of Domitian's own morality laws.

'A penalty has been prescribed against a husband who profits pecuniarily by the adultery of his wife; as well as against one who retains his wife after she has been taken in adultery. Moreover, he who permits his wife to commit this offence holds his marriage in contempt.'[15] This is a stinging rebuke for Domitian from the Augustan laws he set to enforce more stringently on Rome.

Over time the adultery laws became tighter still so that now you didn't have to be the one getting your end away to be prosecuted. 'Anyone who knowingly lends his house to enable debauchery or adultery to be committed there with a matron who is not his wife, or with a male, or who pecuniarily profits by the adultery of his wife, no matter what may be his status, is punished as an adulterer.'[16]

This law gains several amendments that hint at legal wrangling behind the scenes. Clearly some wag had attempted to wriggle out of prosecution by pointing out that he lived in an apartment, hence, 'It is clear that by the term "house" every kind of habitation is meant.'

Having cleared up what a house was, it then became necessary to spell out the meaning of 'his house': 'Anyone who lends the house of a friend is also liable.' You might think this covered every eventuality and underlined the basic principle of not offering a place for adulterous couples to have sex in, but 'Where anyone encourages the commission of debauchery in a field, or in a bath, he should be included in the law.' This strongly hints that at least one enterprising soul was renting out his land for outside fumble fun, as well as recognising that the baths were dens of sexual iniquity and assignation that needed including in the law.

So now we have it, you cannot in any way encourage adultery in the house or apartment that you own, or in a house or apartment that you don't own, or in a place that is not a house or an apartment. Understood? Clearly not, because we get yet another amendment: 'When, however, persons are accustomed to assemble in some house for the purpose of making arrangements to commit adultery, even if it was not committed in that place, still, the owner is considered to have lent his house for the commission of debauchery or adultery, because these offences would not have been perpetrated if these meetings had not taken place.'

Again, underlining the principle that it's the encouragement and facilitation of an illicit liaison that is the crime here. It doesn't matter whether the couple had sex or not – it's the encouragement of it that matters. The entire legal establishment of Rome simultaneously bang their heads on desks.

There are a lot of Roman laws that cover adultery, partly to close loopholes as we have seen, but also to prevent abuses of the law. The way the Roman legal system worked was that anyone could make an accusation against anyone else: they didn't have to be related to the accused or be party to the crime; they needn't have even met the accused.

We see the dark side of this with informers. These were men who spent their days accusing other citizens of crimes – usually treason against the emperor – and then when their hapless victim was convicted, they received a portion of their confiscated estates. Some informers got exceedingly wealthy on this racket.

That there were people trying to exploit the adultery laws for material gain is evident by the thoughtful legal examples that have survived. For example: 'A father-in-law who, in a written accusation filed with the Governor, stated that he accused his daughter-in-law of adultery, preferred to abandon the accusation and obtain her dowry. The question arises whether you think that a scheme of this kind should be permitted.'[17]

The answer in this case was that it should not be permitted because it is shameful to put money above the honour of his household.

Dowry grabbing may be behind this scheme as well, 'If a husband, for the purpose of defaming his wife, provides her with an adulterer, in order that he may catch them.' The ruling here is that in this circumstance both husband and wife will be charged with adultery.

With the coming of Christianity and Christian emperors in the fourth and fifth centuries CE public morals are again taken up in law. Adultery is now punishable not by banishment or by a loss of status, but by actual execution, and a very nasty one at that: the adulterer could expect to be sewn up in a sack and either drowned or burned alive.

Historian Ammianus Marcellinus lists a catalogue of dire punishments dished out to the adulterous: the senator Cethegus was beheaded; Flaviana's clothes were stripped from her during her march to the executioner; Rufina and her lovers, and those who had abetted the adultery, were executed. Marcellinus talks about the 'many' women of high birth who faced death for breaking adultery laws.

Even the emperor's wife was not immune from facing the penalty for adultery as shown by the death of Constantine the Great's wife, Fausta. I say probably, because the execution of Fausta is an affair mired in mystery and intrigue, and raises more questions than it answers.

The mysterious death of the Christian's wife

Flavia Maxima Fausta was the daughter of Emperor Maximian. In 307 CE, in typical Roman fashion, she was married to secure a political alliance between her father, Maximian, and Constantine. Fausta proved to be the perfect dutiful wife. When she discovered her father was plotting against her husband, she told Constantine, putting his security and safety above that of her own family. It was an action that resulted in Maximian's suicide.

Elsewhere she again proved her wifely attributes by popping out six children: three sons and three daughters. Clearly Constantine held her in high esteem since he awarded her the title of Augusta. Then suddenly in 326 CE Fausta is executed. The method of her death somehow involves a hot bath. Zosimus says Constantine caused, 'A bath to be heated to an extraordinary degree, he shut up Fausta in it, and a short time after took her out dead.'[18]

This rather suggests a truly horrible death, being lowered into boiling water. Elsewhere though it is suggested she was suffocated via the hot bath, a method that was used by the Emperor Nero to get rid of his inconvenient wife, Octavia. Either way, Fausta had clearly upset her husband big time. But how?

We might find that the answer is a similarly sudden and unexplained imperial execution a short time before Fausta's death: that of the emperor's son, Crispus. Crispus was the son of Constantine and his first wife, Minerva. Like Fausta, he had been merrily going along his way. He'd been given the highly prestigious title of Caesar in 317 CE and appointed Commander of Gaul. Later, he fought alongside his father in a civil war against Licinius in 324 CE, during which he proved his talent as a general in a decisive naval battle. As a reward, and as proof of Constantine's trust in him, Crispus was assigned some of his father's legions. He married at some point and produced a first grandson for Constantine, an event the emperor celebrated by giving pardons to prisoners.

Overall, Crispus was looking likely successor material, and even appears on the coinage. Until 326 CE when he is abruptly tried and executed. Every single source ties this execution to that of Fausta shortly afterwards, though none of them agrees on the reason, a state of affairs that has tantalised scholars ever since.

Church historian Philostorgius is nicely enigmatic when he says that Crispus was executed due to the machinations of Fausta. Zosimus claims the fault was with Crispus for debauching his stepmother (by 'debauching' Zosimus means rape). Rape is the sort of thing you can well believe Constantine would execute his formally beloved son over. But Zosimus can't quite explain away Fausta's death, relying on the deeply implausible tale that Constantine's mother, Helen, was so devastated by her grandson's death that the emperor killed Fausta so she wouldn't have to be reminded of it.

Zonarus has a different account. 'His [Crispus's] stepmother Fausta was madly in love with him but did not easily get him to go along. She then announced to his father that he [Crispus] loved her and had often attempted to do violence to her. Therefore, Crispus was condemned to death by his father, who believed his wife.'[19]

This ties into Philostorgius' machinations of Fausta and to Zosimus' account of a rape. Put together, we might theorise that Fausta, perhaps with her three sons and their succession in mind, concocted a tale of Crispus raping her or otherwise being inappropriate. Crispus was tried and executed, presumably under the adultery laws. Later, Constantine uncovers Fausta's deception and executes her too.

That there is something to the rumours is proven by the fact that even when Fausta's three sons became emperor after Constantine's death they did not lift the *damnatio memoriae* on their mother or try in any way to redeem her memory. We can theorise, but we can never know and the whole event remains tantalisingly shadowy.

To conclude, adultery was something that Romans were so extremely concerned about that they introduced legislation and ever harsher punishments to those found guilty of the offence. That the legislation was tinkered with repeatedly suggests it wasn't terribly effective.

At various points emperors found themselves in situations where they themselves, or their families, were contravening adultery legislation, leaving them with quite the dilemma. Although Augustus cracked down on the adulterous liaisons of the women in his household, he did nothing to curb his own. Domitian tried to stick to the letter of the law that he was avidly promoting by banishing his adulterous wife, but he couldn't bear to be without her. The only emperor we find actively sticking to their laws is Constantine in executing both his wife and her lover (we think).

Chapter 13

Homosexuality

This is a very poorly titled chapter for in ancient Rome there was no such thing as homosexuality; there isn't even a word in Latin for it. Which is probably confusing you right now since we have so far covered Mark Antony's alleged career as a rent boy, Augustus getting adopted by Julius Caesar by way of sexual favours and that bloke who scrawled on a wall in Pompeii that he'd given up women and was now all about penetrating men's behinds. Not to mention that mysterious hand gesture used by Clodius to taunt Pompey and others which appears to be used as a devastating comment on their masculinity. Surely that's all about being homosexual?

So, what's the score? Yes, there were same sex relationships in ancient Rome and plenty of them but there were very different societal rules governing them. Romans did not fit themselves into exclusive pots of who they fancied, they did not describe themselves as heterosexual or homosexual. Rather they had words that described the sexual act they were partaking in and how they were participating in it. Some of these words we met in our first chapter such as *futuo* – to penetrate a vagina – *pedico* – to penetrate an anus – *irrumare* – to penetrate forcibly a mouth. The gender was not important, the sexual act was, and very particularly what role you played in it.

We saw this play out in our chapter looking at *virtus* and the danger Roman youths faced in protecting it. Also, in our chapter on language, where we saw that the very worst insults you could throw at a Roman male involved him being penetrated in his mouth. The graffiti from Pompeii and Herculaneum is riddled with a huge number of *fellators*, such as poor Cosmus who, because of a singular volcanic eruption is forever immortalised as: 'Cosmos is a big queer and a cocksucker with his legs wide open.'

Real Roman men, men with *virtus*, were forever the penetrator, never the penetrated. There were words for the latter; *pathicus* is the most brutally direct, it meant one who submits to anal sex. There was no mistaking the accusation there, but there were also other words that were not so direct such as *mollis*, meaning soft, and *effeminatus*, which doesn't really need translating. Other terms used include *cinaedus* and *catamite*, both have their origin in dancing and particularly the dancers who would wriggle their buttocks about.

There is a lot of scroll space given in Roman literature on how to spot one of these soft men or *cinadae*. The clothing apparently is a dead giveaway. Scipio Aemilianus, who describes Publius Africanus as having shaven eyebrows, a plucked beard and wearing a leotard, concludes, 'Does anyone doubt about him, that he did the same thing that *cinaedi* do?'[1]

Seneca singles out Augustus' right-hand man, Maecenas, as effeminate because he 'always paraded through the city with a flowing tunic.'[2] Caligula's dress sense similarly gives away his predilections, 'He often appeared in public in embroidered cloaks covered with precious stones, with a long-sleeved tunic and bracelets; sometimes in silk and in a woman's robe; now in slippers or buskins.'[3]

The walk was another giveaway, again something Seneca attributes to Maecenas. 'We know how he walked,' he says, and then refuses to elaborate how and what about it made it effeminate. Juvenal is similarly opaque, mentioning the effeminate male 'who admits his affliction in his looks and his walk.'[4]

I guess we are all imaging at this point they are referring to a mince: an effeminate man, in a long tunic mincing. Let us add to the stereotype this from Cicero on Gabinius, '[He] had carefully-dressed hair, and perfumed fringes of curls, and anointed and carefully-rouged cheeks.'[5]

Juvenal has the full checklist of what an effeminate male looks like: 'One man has blackened his eyebrows, moistened with soot, Extends them with slanting pencil, and flutters his eyelids, While applying the make-up; another drinks from a phallus-shaped glass, his bouffant hair filling a gilded hair-net, dressed in a chequered blue or a yellow-green satin.'[6]

So far so obvious, but a mincing walk, a fully made-up face and wearing a dress were not the only signs of a *cinaedus*. Another way to spot an effeminate male was to look for the very opposite, a manly male, 'Find some uncouth, rough-chinned philosopher who's always harping on the days that were! You'll find one; but that grim old Roman set is riddled with queers,'[7] scoffs Martial. Juvenal has a similar tale of men hiding their predilections behind hairy arms and bodies and upright views.

All of which again highlights just what a surveillance society Rome was. Not only were your walk, your tunic, your beard, your voice, your everything constantly being scrutinised for the barest whiff of softness, but also your walk, your tunic, your beard, your voice, your everything was being scrutinised for a suspicious lack of softness that might prove you are effeminate and partaking in passive anal sex. Being a Roman man must have been stressful.

The *pathicus*, though, was not exclusively into men, not homosexual in the way we think about the word. Rather he was, in Roman eyes, a sexual deviant who might well be indulging with both men and women. Juvenal has this warning for husbands about that eunuch in their house, 'A hair-netted adulterer he'll paint his eyelids with mascara, and strut around with his saffron gown undone. You should be the more suspicious.'[8]

All emperors who were noted as submitting to anal sex, such as Caligula, of whom Valerius Catullus said that he had 'buggered the emperor and quite worn himself out in the process,'[9] were also prolific lovers of women. Caligula, for instance, was said to have inspected the wives of his dinner guests and taken away the ones he most fancied for a quick shag before returning them to their rightful owner.

The deviancy at the heart of this is that the *cinaedus* or *pathicus*, or whatever you want to call him, is a passive creature giving pleasure to others: he is not a do-er, he is inactive. Being a do-er is what Rome and being a Roman man is all about. Doing was service to the State, doing is what created their empire. If you are engaged in copious amounts of sex with all genders you are inactive, not doing, and so neglecting your service to the State.

Most of these accusations of being soft, womanly and submitting to anal sex are just that, accusations: it's rhetoric with a sharp pointed end. But all these insults tell us something about the nature of what was taboo in ancient Rome, and being penetrated by another man was so unacceptable as to make you suspect in the eyes of all of society. Something the Emperor Vitellius could certainly attest to. He spent his youth on Capri during the time of the wildest rumours spread about Tiberius, which earnt Vitellius the nickname 'Spintria' meaning pervert. We are told this nickname stuck to him for the rest of his life.

The combination of this taboo and Romans not categorising people exclusively by gender preference means that you will be extremely hard pressed to find any examples in all Roman history of consenting adult males in a long-term romantic/sexual relationship. There simply aren't any. I say consenting and adult particularly, because as I said earlier, there were same sex relationships in ancient Rome, but they operated according to very different criteria, as we shall now explore further.

Serving the master

The important caveat in Roman society is that the taboo of being penetrated applies only to freeborn men. We saw this in the Lex Scantinia. The 'shameful' acts that were prosecutable were only those perpetrated against free men and women; slaves, ex-slaves and those tainted with *infamia* were fair game. As Seneca neatly summarises, 'Sexual passivity in a free man is a crime, for a slave a necessity, for a freed slave a duty.'[10]

That slaves were used for sexual services by their owners is imbedded in Roman society. 'Still, I was my master's favourite for fourteen years. No disgrace in obeying your master's orders. Well, I used to amuse my mistress too. You know what I mean; I say no more, I am not a conceited man.'[11] So says the freedman Timalchio in Petronius's *Satyricon*.

'He must remain awake throughout the night, dividing his time between his master's drunkenness and his lust,' says Seneca on the plight of many male slaves. Horace, neatly and somewhat horrifyingly, summarises why sex with slaves is preferable to that with free women, they are easy:

> Do you ask for a golden cup when you're dying
> Of thirst? Do you scorn all but peacock, or turbot
> When you're starving? When your prick swells, then,
> And a young slave girl or boy's nearby you could take
> At that instant, would you rather burst with desire?
> Not I: I love the sexual pleasure that's easy to get.[12]

The names given to some slaves were a deliberate cruelty and a constant reminder of their duties. We find names that translate as sexy, hot legs, desire, beloved, pleasure, kiss. Slaves were lacking in any control over their bodies. Cato the Elder deciding that his male slaves were more troublesome if sexually frustrated gave them each a female slave to sate themselves with. Neither male nor female slave would have had any say in this. Nor did the chosen slave partner in Horace's poem quoted above: Horace's pleasure is paramount; the nearby slave girl or boy does not even enter into consideration.

This goes a long way to explaining the social stigma held against freedmen. The contempt freedmen are held in by the likes of Tacitus, even when they are holding high positions, likely has its roots in a disgust at what services they are assumed to have performed in their previous status. And not just as slaves, for even after being manumitted, freedman were still beholden to their former master, as was stated in law, 'A freedman is compelled to support his patron, if he is in want, by means of gifts, presents, and services, to the extent of his means.'[13]

The word 'services' is nicely ambiguous and undoubtedly included sexual services in a lot of cases, and we do have a number of examples of freedmen being involved sexually with their ex-masters.

Imperial favourites

The freedmen we have the most information about are those attached to the imperial household and it is clear from our sources that they too were involved in providing 'services' to their ex-master, the emperor.

During Nero's time both slave and freed are sucked into the emperor's peculiar sex games: 'He at last devised a kind of game, in which, covered with the skin of some wild animal, he was let loose from a cage and attacked the private parts of men and women, who were bound to stakes, and when he had sated his mad lust, was dispatched by his freedman Doryphorus.'[14]

Not that it makes this scenario any less extreme, but I believe we can translate 'attacked the private parts' as performed oral sex on. Doryphorus too is in possession of a name that translates as 'spear man', which makes you wonder whether Suetonius is making a double entendre here, not least because Doryphorus is given the name Pythagorus in other sources.

Pythagorus/Doryphorus has the key part in another one of Nero's sex games where he plays the groom to Nero's bride: 'he stooped to marry himself to one of that filthy herd, by name Pythagoras, with all the forms of regular wedlock. The bridal veil was put over the emperor; people saw the witnesses of the ceremony, the wedding dower, the couch and the nuptial torches; everything in a word was plainly visible, which, even when a woman weds darkness hides.'[15]

After the ceremony Pythagorus performed his conjugal duties, Nero giving the performance of his lifetime by '[imitating] the cries and lamentations of a maiden being deflowered.'[16]

What can we make of this? Firstly, that Nero had far too much time on his hands that surely could have been put to better use. Secondly, it's all a game, a bit of sexual role play.

With such stories circulating we might start to understand why the historians of the day, such as Tacitus, have such an engrained snobbery towards imperial freedman. Nero's 'games' were odd enough to warrant recording, but there must have been plenty of other 'games' with freedmen that were not.

Another tale of an emperor and his freedman which is worth examining is that of Vitellius and Asiaticus. Vitellius is depicted by our sources as owning the very worst of attributes: cruelty, gluttony, greed and that most Roman of offences, being under the thrall of lesser social classes, 'he regulated the greater part of his rule wholly according to the advice and whims of the commonest of actors and chariot-drivers, and in particular of his freedman Asiaticus.'[17]

Asiaticus is portrayed in our sources, much like the powerful trio of freedmen from Claudius' day, as being entirely undeserving of holding the position he did. Or as Tacitus describes him, '[A] servile, shameful creature, who owed his popularity to his wicked arts.'[18]

The wicked arts Tacitus refers to are sexual, not just because of the overall assumption that freedmen would have been used sexually by their masters but also because of Asiaticus' own back story. We are told he was Vitellius' favourite bed partner until Asiaticus ran away.

Vitellius happens to stumble across his runaway slave working as a barman in the coastal town of Puetoli. Asiaticus was put in chains and taken back, where he found himself back in Vitellius' favour, at least for a while. But then Asiaticus annoys Vitellius with his insolence and is sold to a gladiator troop. On the very day Asiaticus was to make his debut as a gladiator, Vitellius swept in and brought him back. Asiaticus is freed and serves in Vitellius' administration, making a tidy fortune for himself.

This is what Tacitus considers a servile and shameful person, someone whose past is so dubious that they shouldn't be allowed to serve in a public position serving the state – or benefitting from it in any way.

We view this from a different perspective without the baggage of Roman cultural expectations and through a prism of human rights. What do we see? We see a slave abused sexually by his master from childhood, who could take no more abuse and ran away. This is no rash decision; the punishments for runaway slaves were dire and they would be constantly terrified of being caught and returned.

Which is what happens to Asiaticus when Vitellius finds him by the coast. Then he's back in favour and by favour we can assume bedroom favours are involved, until he annoys Vitellius and is sold. That he is sold to a gladiatorial troop only underpins the cruelty of Vitellius, as does the sudden rescue. Was that the plan the whole time: to frighten Asiaticus so that he knows his place and that he can be sold at any moment?

He's freed by Vitellius but still tied to his abuser. That abuser becomes emperor and Asiaticus uses the opportunity to enrich himself or perhaps pay himself properly for his job in the administration. It's open to interpretation and we have no way of knowing which is the more valid version. Likely Tacitus, a man of the era, has it right the whole time.

Vitellius' predecessor as emperor, Galba, was another one who had a long-standing relationship with one of his freedmen. Galba's preference was for sturdy, hard men. His freedman, Icelus, apparently fell into this category. When Icelus brought news of Nero's suicide to Galba, the new emperor greeted his freedman with fond kisses and dragged him off for celebratory sex.

Like Asiaticus, Icelus serves in an imperial administration, and also like Asiaticus he is portrayed as a grabbing, greedy immoral man: 'Icelus has stolen more than all that a Polyclitus and a Vatinius and an Aegialus squandered,' sneers Tacitus.

There is perhaps lurking under Tacitus' disdain a realisation that freedmen had an advantage over the freeborn, in that they were already close to an emperor and could offer sex as a way of advancement. There is nowhere in Tacitus any understanding or acknowledgment that a freedman might have legitimately gained his role by being good at his job. All who are mentioned are greedy, grasping and entirely unworthy.

Although the caveat here is that Galba's two other advisors, Vinius and Laco, both freeborn, get as bad press as Icelus. The difference in their status, however, is underlined by their deaths when Galba is overthrown in a coup. Vinius and Galba are killed in an all-out massacre that took place in the Forum on 15 January 69 CE. Laco was arrested and banished to an island, later to be bumped off by an assassin sent by Galba's successor, Otho. Icelus is arrested and publicly crucified, something that as a freedman he should have been safe from. A public death on display is a clear demonstration of what happens to uppity ex-slaves, they could never escape their past.

As we've noted before, a sexual relationship with a freedman did not make a Roman homosexual. Nero, Vitellius and Galba were, or had been, married. Suetonius and our other sources see no contradiction in this double gender sex life, and where entanglements with freedmen are mentioned it's to highlight a deficiency in the emperor: the story of Asiaticus shows up Vitellius' cruelty that is evident everywhere in his reign; Galba made Icelus too much of a favourite and showed up his blindness to his aides' corruption; and Nero's increasingly elaborate role play games demonstrated his loosening grip on reality, which played a major part in his downfall.

Boys

'If someone allowed me to carry on kissing those honeyed eyes of yours, I would kiss them right on to three hundred thousand nor would I ever think I was going to be sated.'[19] So says Catullus rather touchingly. But the subject of this poem is not his mistress, Lesbia, rather it is addressed to Juventius, meaning young man.

It is not the only poem Catullus writes to Juventius: 'Honeyed Juventius, while you were playing, I stole from you a little kiss sweeter than sweet ambrosia.'[20] In fact, for all his honeyed eyes and sweet lips, Juventius was quite as troublesome to Catullus as his mistress, Lesbia.

Just as Lesbia played cruelly with Catullus' affections (see the chapter Love Hurts, for the full heart-breaking story) Juventius is also the lover of a certain Aurelius. Catullus' response to this competition is very typical: he threatens to anally rape Aurelius with a radish and a mullet. The fact that there is no difference in how Catullus treats Juventius and Lesbia in his poems is telling: there was no distinction between sleeping with a woman or a boy to Catullus.

Love poet Tibullus interjects poems despairing about his mistress, Delia, with ones despairing about Marathus in a poem entitled 'The Love of Boys': 'Alas how Marathus torments me with love's delay!'[21]

Martial is not averse to boys either, 'I'd rather put up with these haughty, querulous, blood minded naughty boys than be married to some bitch who makes me miserably rich.'[22] Even the Emperor Trajan, we are told by Cassius Dio, was devoted to boys, although we are assured it was not excessive. It is considered by Suetonius a noteworthy, recordable fact about the Emperor Claudius that he liked women with an excessive passion, but boys and men left him cold.

To conclude, love affairs with boys were considered both normal and acceptable in ancient Rome. The question lingers, though. Hanging over every declaration of love, every honeyed phrase, what do we mean by 'boy'?

It's an uncomfortable question for us living in the twenty-first century and it hangs like a dark cloud over Catullus' admittedly beautiful poems to Juventius: how young was that young man? Are these honeyed kisses being bestowed on a child by an adult man? There is another uncomfortable question here too – where are the poems dedicated to adult men by adult men? The answer in this case is straightforward, there aren't any. I'm afraid we need to unpack what can only be described as an unsavoury aspect of ancient Roman society.

They are sometimes described as *pullus*, meaning young chicken. It was an apt word, the transformation from a soft, fluffy chick to a fully feathered adult bird is quite a transformative one, and so it was for the Roman boy moving from being a child to an adult. They are sometimes called *puer delicatas* – delicate boys.

In poetry they are described as soft and smooth. The smooth is important for it denotes a lack of facial hair and the appearance of the facial hair was the moment that a *puer* stopped being an acceptable sexual partner. These were pre-adolescent boys, but, importantly, they were slaves. The *stuprum* laws protected the chastity of freeborn boys, but slaves had no such protections.

A list of job titles from the imperial palace under Augustus has amongst the shoemakers and silver keepers the job of delicate boy. These delicate boys had their own beautician to take care of their appearance. The Emperor Titus kept his own harem of boys and eunuchs, although we are told by Suetonius that he gave up some of his favourite boys on becoming emperor, unlike Trajan.

In ancient Athens and some of the other Greek city states, relationships between men and boys had been romanticised. This was a courting between an older man, known as an *erastes*, and a boy, the *eromenos*. The *erastes* was expected to teach his *eromenos* what it took to be a man, to educate him and act as a role model. It was also a connection that would likely serve the *eromenos* well in his adult life. There were strict cultural norms around how this courting took place and how each partner would behave. It should also be noted that the sexual side of this relationship stopped short of sodomy, rather the adult male would ejaculate between the grasped thighs of the boy.

Such relationships feature heavily on black and red earthenware vases from the time, with the *erastes* always featured with a beard. The nature of ancient Greek pederasty can appear soft at first glance, romanticised, full of images of beautiful, perfectly formed young men. In comparison, Roman pederasty is described brutally and anatomically in the likes of Martial. But the Romans were horrified at Greek pederasty. It was abominable to them, because the boys involved were all freeborn and high born. Freeborn boys in Rome were protected by law from such abuses and they couldn't understand Greek pederasty any more than we can today.

This objectification of boys made them a highly prized commodity in the slave markets; they could be worth more than an adult male slave based on their beauty alone. The slave dealers being canny businessmen had methods of prolonging the usefulness of their stock, a mixture of hyacinth bulbs and sweet wine was said to prevent the onset of puberty, particularly beard growth. The most successful way of preventing puberty and maintaining that beard-free soft cheek, however, was castration.

Seneca talks about wine boys, forced to pretend to still be boys long after they'd reached maturity. 'He is kept beardless by having his hair smoothed away or plucked out by the roots.'[23] Even as adults, slaves were often addressed as boy, infantilising them but also keeping them open for sex.

The favourite – Antinous

The most famous same-sex relationship in Roman history is that of Hadrian with Antinous. 'During a journey on the Nile he lost Antinous, his favourite.' So says the *Historia Augusta* on Antinous and this is all they have to say about him.

They are not alone. Search through the sources and you will find scant mention of Hadrian's great favourite, Antinous. He doesn't appear to hold any key position in Hadrian's administration. True, he follows the emperor on his tour of the provinces, but there is no mention of him having any kind of role during this. There aren't any anecdotes recounted of their love affair, not even any dodgy sexual practices as with Nero and his freedmen, nor any comment on how the Empress Sabina felt about the young man. There aren't any stories at all on Antinous, save for the one mentioning his death. He is almost entirely unnoteworthy for our sources to bother recording. That they don't feel compelled to mention Hadrian's favourite is perhaps illustrative of how common it was for an emperor to have a favourite boy.

So why am I mentioning him at all? Because although Antinous in life barely dents the pages of history, in death he becomes something else entirely.

In the mid-first century CE, a Greek by the name of Pausanias was pottering around Greece undertaking an extremely useful assignment: he was writing a guidebook aimed at tourists which detailed all the things they should see during their holiday. Pausanias' guide to Greece is a treasure trove of information on what archaeological sites were standing in the first century CE and the stories behind them. As well as giving us an insight on what travelling Romans would find interesting, and some handy hints for our tourists such as the difficulty of the terrain for walking.

In his chapter on the Arcadia area, Pausainas has this titbit for us: 'There is a building in the gymnasium of Mantineia containing statues of Antinous, and remarkable for the stones with which it is adorned, and especially so for its pictures. Most of them are portraits of Antinous, who is made to look just like Dionysus.'[24]

Mantineia was not alone in being in possession of statues of Antinous. There must have been images of him everywhere in the empire, for the surprising thing about Hadrian's generally unnoteworthy favourite is that there are more surviving depictions of him than of many emperors.

There are eighteen surviving statues of Antinous, fifteen busts, fifty-three heads and he features in two reliefs. These were found in such disparate locations as Syria, Italy, Greece, North Africa, Spain, Egypt, Syria and even Britain. Why so many?

Firstly, obviously he meant a lot to Hadrian. When Antinous died Hadrian was said to have 'cried like a woman'.[25] Cassius Dio states that Hadrian honoured Antinous because of his love for him, before throwing in a massive 'or because', which we will explore shortly. Honoured Antinous certainly was and not just as statues. There was the city Hadrian founded in Egypt on the spot where the boy died, naming it Antinoöpolis after his lost love. This is highly unusual: if Romans were going to name a settlement it would be after themselves (see Constantinople), not some lowly attendant.

But it gets even more extreme, for we are also told that Hadrian made Antinous a god. Where Pausanias is describing the statues of Antinous in his guidebook he is doing so outside a temple to this new god. Pausanias tells us, 'The Emperor established his worship in Mantineia also; mystic rites are celebrated in his honour each year, and games every four years.'

Mantineia was far from alone in being in possession of a temple to Antinous. Sites identified with worship of Antinous have been found in the Greek cities of Eleusis, Delphi, Corinth and Symrna, also in Turkey, Egypt and Italy. That Antinous was deified despite having no familiar connection with the imperial family is highly unusual. The effort Hadrian put into venerating his memory and setting up games in his honour is highly unusual. What was going on?

Antinous, we are told, was from the city of Bithynium in the province of Bithynia, in modern-day Turkey. At some point in his life he joined Hadrian's travelling entourage. At another point he took part in a lion hunt with the emperor. Then towards the end of 130 CE Antinous drowned in the river Nile. That is it. That is all we know.

However, from his many portraits we know at least what he looked like: shaggy hair, contemplative expression, a six-pack and a squeezably pert bottom. In short, Antinous was drop-dead gorgeous. He was also visibly still a boy, most likely in his mid-teens at the time of his death, while Hadrian was fifty-four years old.

We can romanticise it all we like, the utter devastation and grief of Hadrian recreating Antinous' image across the world so that he could never be forgotten, Hadrian partaking of 'Greek love' being a mentor to the young Antinous, but he was still a fifty-four-year-old man having a sexual relationship with a teenager who was not in a position to refuse. An affair, which, as we have seen, would have tainted Antinous throughout his adult life.

One of the many theories behind his mysterious death is that Antinous committed suicide, either because he'd reached his limit as a sex object or that Hadrian wanted to continue the liaison despite Antinous having reached manhood – a state that would have cast the ultimate disgrace on them both.

Alternatively, Antinous sacrificed himself in a religious ritual to improve Hadrian's health or was sacrificed against his will for similar reasons. Antinous' death clearly caused much talk, because apparently Hadrian felt compelled to defend himself in his autobiography (long since lost). But there is no ultimate solution to this mystery, or the mystery of why Antinous was so special. As with the other slaves, freedmen and boys mentioned in this chapter, we do not have his voice. We have no clue how Antinous, or Pythagorus or Asiasticus felt about their relationship with an emperor, we have no idea whether they were willing lovers or compelled by the lowliness of their positions. This lack of information matters.

Legal matters

The law protected freeborn boys from a shameful act being perpetrated against them under the Lex Scantinia, Domitian added to these protections by banning the prostitution of boys, earning him this breathless compliment from Martial, 'Before this, Caesar, you were loved by boys, and youths, and old men; now infants also love you.'[26]

Alexander Severus decided to make a moral stand and as well as forcing women of ill repute to become prostitutes he also deports male prostitutes from Rome. He would also have banned this form of prostitution altogether we are told, 'but he feared that such a prohibition would merely convert an evil recognized by the state into a vice practised in private – for men when driven on by passion are more apt to demand a vice which is prohibited.'[27]

That job fell to Philip the Arab, who, nine years later, banned male prostitution entirely. Although evidently this did not stamp out the practise entirely since at the Christian Council of Elvira in 306 CE it was decided that, 'Parents and other Christians who give up their children to sexual abuse are selling others' bodies, and if they do so or sell their own bodies, they shall not receive communion even at death.'[28]

However, this disquiet over same-sex relations starts to grow and extend outside of prostitution, particularly when Christianity began to spread as a religion. At the Council of Ancyra in 314 CE we find communion refused to those guilty of what are called 'bestial lusts'. This is followed in the next canon by those guilty of bestiality and lepers who have knowingly infected others.

The language used to describe same-sex relations hardens. An edict issued by two of Constantine the Great's sons in 342 CE makes this clear, 'We do not endure that the city of Rome, the mother of all virtues and manly excellence to be the contamination of effeminised shame in a man.'

This edict very particularly is concerned with men playing the woman's role in sex, that is, being the passive partner: 'Therefore all those who practise sexual debauchery by condemning their manly body that they refashioned in a womanly way through yielding.' In the previous centuries this was an accusation that was hurled about in political speeches or made fun of by Martial in poems, but in this era things have turned distinctly nasty. Now those accused of being penetrated are hit not with a witty riposte by the likes of Cicero, or an offensive nickname, but rather, 'the avenging powers of flame'. They are burnt alive in other words.

The same strongly worded language is found in the law: 'We order the statutes to arise, the laws to be armed with an avenging sword, that those infamous persons who are now, or who hereafter may be, guilty may be subjected to exquisite punishment.'[29]

The Justinian code of laws put together in the sixth century talks of 'certain men, seized by diabolical incitement practice among themselves the most disgraceful lusts, and act contrary to nature.' Interestingly, these disgraceful lusts are described as a danger to the city and state in much the same way as women's sexual behaviour.

These punishments are still very much aimed at the passive male in homosexual sex, but the language is notably harsher than in earlier era. Combined with the extreme punishments meted out to anyone convicted, this truly was the end of any kind of toleration. Although it should be noted that one of the emperors who put his name to that edict targeting those practising sexual debauchery was himself accused of having the same vices. Constans II, the son of Constantine the Great, is accused in sources of scandalous behaviour with handsome barbarian hostages.

Lesbians

Like most of this book so far, this chapter has been all about men, their sexuality and their desires. That, unfortunately, is the nature of a patriarchal society: women don't much feature in anyone's concerns. Not surprisingly, there are few mentions of same-sex relations between women, but they are mentioned. The word used for lesbians is *tribades*, which comes from the Greek *tribo*, meaning 'I rub'.

For dream interpreter Artemidorus, sex between women was categorised as an act contrary to nature; it appears after a whole section on the meaning behind a dreaming of having sex with your mother. If you dream of penetrating another woman, according to Artemidorus, you will pursue matters that come to nothing. Which is an interesting insight into what they thought of the worth of lesbian sex.

Juvenal makes a reference to Tullia and Maura, who after a night out stop at the Temple of Chastity for a wee break and then 'take it in turns to ride and squirm under the moon.'[30]

Martial writes about a certain Bassa, who he has never seen hanging out with men. He'd assumed she was a virtuous Lucretia, but:

> You were an active humper all the time.
> You improvised, by rubbing cunts together,
> And using that bionic clit of yours
> To counterfeit the thrusting of a male.[31]

Bassa is dominant here, playing the man with her oversized clitoris acting as a penis. Another poem of Martial features the extremely masculine Philaenis. Martial ticks off the ways in which she is like a man: she goes to the gym to play handball and wrestle, she builds up a sweat, she drinks to excess and then vomits it up in time for dinner, she eats to excess and yes, she fucks to excess too. 'After all this, it's time to fuck. Pricks she won't suck; she thinks it's sissy, but gobbles up the cracks of girls.'[32]

Martial has her sleeping with eleven girls a day and also buggering boys. She is 'hornier than a married man', he tells us. Aside from the cunnilingus at the end, Philaenis reads like a pastiche of a hyper-masculine Roman male who sleeps with both boys and women, eats, drinks, exercises and is all in all a bit of a bore. Bassa by comparison sleeps only with women, which puzzles Martial, 'Only the Sphinx could read this riddle right: With males renounced, adultery can flourish.'

As well as rubbing, lesbian sex was assumed to involve acts of penetration with dildos, or as Lucian calls them 'cunningly contrived instruments of lechery, those mysterious monstrosities devoid of seed.'[33] Which sex toy manufactures should really use in their marketing. Although there are no Roman images of women with dildos, it features repeatedly on ancient Greek vases.

Lucian makes the case for allowing women to sleep with women, 'Come now, epoch of the future, legislator of strange pleasures, devise fresh paths for male lusts, but bestow the same privilege upon women, and let them have intercourse with each other just as men do.'

Affairs between women did occur, despite the lack of space given to them in sources. Amongst the many love spells found is one to bind two women together. Sophia desperately wants Gorgonia, 'By means of the corpse-demon inflame the heart, the liver, and the spirit of Gorgonia [...] with love and affection for Sophia.'[34]

The double theme running through commentary on lesbianism is that it is not natural and that it poses a threat to men, which is typical for Rome. Let's talk about the men again!

Chapter 14

Undesirable Partners

We have looked at what were acceptable sexual practises and partners in ancient Rome, examining the legality of adultery and homosexuality along the way. But aside from married women and freeborn boys, there were other classes of people in Rome who were deemed unsuitable partners and who suffered both cultural and legal constraints as a result, though at the same time they might also be the most popular and famous person in Rome. It's in no way a straightforward tale, but then nothing is in ancient Rome!

Breaking the class barrier

Rome was a very class-based society. At the very top were the Senatorial class who numbered 600 men and their families: this was Rome's ruling class and the one from which nearly all public magistrates came. To maintain the dignity of this class the Augustan morality laws had placed restrictions on who they could marry.

One such restriction was this one: 'Senators, as well as their children, are forbidden to marry their freedwomen.'[1] There was nothing, however, in the law that forbade relationships with a freedwoman and these did occur in the highest of circles. Some, though, were distinctly unromantic, such as this winning strategy for gaining entrance to Nero's inner circle by future emperor Otho, 'he pretended love for an influential freedwoman of the court, although she was an old woman and almost decrepit, that he might more effectually win her favour.'[2]

In law there was no impediment to these relationships and even some freedoms, for example, the Augustan laws on adultery did not apply. A freedwoman with a conviction for adultery was not prevented from entering a relationship with a man, provided she did not marry him (which she couldn't anyway if he were of senatorial or equestrian class). Another act pertains, 'Where a freedwoman is living in concubinage with her patron, she can leave him without his consent, and unite with another man, either in matrimony or in concubinage.'[3]

The only restrictions applied in those cases were that the freedwoman mistress had to be over twelve years old, as was also standard for the freeborn.

A love story across the divide: Vespasian and Antonia Caenis

This is the love story of an imperial freedwoman and an emperor. Antonia Caenis had been a secretary to the Emperor Claudius' mother, Antonia.[4] Titus Flavius Vespasian was your bog-standard Roman male trying to make it in politics. At some point the two met and began a relationship.

At the start of this relationship it was Caenis who was probably the more powerful. Vespasian was from an inconsequential family, Caenis on the other hand had a wealth of imperial connections and influence. Like Otho's freedwoman, she probably would have used that influence to promote Vespasian. I say probably, because we will never know for sure, but Vespasian's career did prosper.

Despite Caenis' position at the centre of court and despite her many excellent qualities (Cassius Dio calls her a remarkable woman), the law was clear; Caenis' status as a freedwoman meant they could not marry. Instead Vespasian married Flavia Domitilla, who although not from an especially distinguished family was considered suitable, legal marriage material. They probably married around the year 38 CE, because in 39 CE their first child, the future Emperor Titus, was born. They had two more children, a daughter, Domitilla, and another future emperor, Domitian.

During this marriage it appears Caenis and Vespasian called off their relationship. There was no reason why they should have, there would have been no shame attached to Vespasian in keeping her as his mistress, provided he was not too excessive in his regard for her. We might speculate, therefore, that it was Caenis who put an end to it.[5]

Vespasian never forgot her though, because when his wife died (in the 60s CE most likely) we are told he rekindled his romance with Caenis and treated her as his lawful wife, even after he was emperor. Cassius Dio tells us, rather sweetly, that: 'Vespasian took such excessive delight in her.'[6]

She seems to have played some role in state business acting as an intermediary for Vespasian, selling off positions such as governorships and priesthoods, and then, presumably, funnelling the money back to the emperor. Vespasian could thus simultaneously improve the condition of the treasury while appearing free of corruption. She certainly amassed a great wealth during this time, we are told.

Vespasian may have treated her as his wife, but she was not empress and whatever role she might have played behind the scenes in the administration she does not, unlike Vespasian's late wife, Flavia Domitilla, appear on the official coinage or any other portraiture. We are told that Vespasian's younger son, Domitian, refused to greet Caenis with a kiss but instead held out his hand to her, perhaps as a reminder of her place and inferior social status.

Caenis stayed by Vespasian's side until her death in 74 CE. An inscription dedicated to her confirms her position as the emperor's official companion: 'This funerary altar to Antonia Caenis, mistress of Vespasian and freedwoman of Antonia Minor, daughter of Octavia and Marc Antony, was set up by her freedman on the estate of her villa on the Via Nomentana in Rome.'

Vespasian himself died in 79 CE. It's a terribly romantic story: the clever ex-slave at the centre of court; the humble but aspiring well-bred young man falling deeply in love, but forbidden by law to marry; then the family pressure that was surely placed on Vespasian to marry the right sort of girl and produce heirs; the undoubtedly desperately emotional scene where Caenis breaks off their relationship, possibly, we may speculate, to force Vespasian to do the proper thing and marry Flavia. Then we have the years they spent apart yearning for each other, and the joyous reunion (when Flavia was suitably dead for a time). What an emotional rollercoaster! I won't ruin the tale by pointing out that after Caenis' death Vespasian took up with 'several' concubines. We'll pretend that never happened.

Nero and Acte

Another emotionally draining romance between an emperor and a freedwoman is that of Nero and Acte. Nero fell deeply in love with Acte, more than his wife, Octavia, who he was not so fond of (and later had killed), and soon she was his constant companion.

Nero had a great plan to deal with the legal aspect: he convinced (aka bribed with money) two consuls to swear that Acte was of royal birth, thus making it perfectly legal for him to wed her. However, a marriage did not take place, legally or otherwise, between Nero and Acte. This was most likely because of pressure applied from Nero's mother, Agrippina, who objected strongly to the relationship. This objection seems less to do with Acte's status as a freedwoman and more to do with her influence on Nero. Mother was being pushed out of the picture and did not take it well.

Agrippina's methods of removing this unwanted influence on her son was to first attack his associates (or unsuitable friends as we might otherwise call them). When that didn't work, or he constant nagging, she reminded him, 'It was I who made you emperor.'[7] The hint being that: a) Nero should be damn grateful to her, and b) she could make him an ex-emperor just as easily.

We can take the very public poisoning of Nero's stepbrother and likely heir, Britannicus, at an imperial banquet shortly afterwards as the emperor's reply to his mother. Presumably he was too scared to tell her face to face what he thought about her threats.

In talking about Nero and his mother we have neglected the key protagonist of this tale, Acte. But then she gets scant mention in our sources. There is nothing about her looks or her character or anything that she and Nero did together. She is enigmatically mysterious, the freedwoman who stole an emperor's heart.

Nero did not marry her, so perhaps Agrippina's devious tactics worked: this time (a little later her nagging would lead her son to have her killed). But there is evidence that Nero and Acte's relationship may have continued.

After Nero's suicide in 68 CE his old nurse and Acte are both present at the entombment of his ashes. Suetonius refers to Acte in this context as Nero's mistress, so perhaps she had been there the whole time in the background. Acte, unlike Antonia Caenis, had no public role as Nero's consort or in the administration in any way, but her presence at his funeral, one of only two people to be there, shows the depths of her loyalty and affection towards the late emperor. Pretty much everyone else had abandoned Nero when his fortunes started to ebb.

Although marriage between the highest two classes and freed people was forbidden, relationships, as we have seen, between them were acceptable. There is no personal criticism directed towards Acte and Caenis in our sources, nor really towards Nero and Vespasian for choosing them. Had Nero succeeded in his efforts to marry Acte we might have seen a different take on a relationship that would then have overstepped the mark of decent behaviour. But he did not, so we do not.

Beneath the senatorial and equestrian rank we find evidence of marriages between freed people and Roman citizens. But there was a group of people that all freeborn Romans were forbidden to marry, whether they be a senator living in a large villa on the Caelian Hill or a carpenter barely making ends meet in an overcrowded apartment building in the rundown Aventine area: the *infames*.

Infamia roughly translates as lacking in reputation and is linked with those nebulous Roman concepts of honour and *virtus*. Someone tainted with *infamia* was someone without *virtus* and who could never hope to have any. This was a significant stigma and it set them apart from the rest of society.

You could buy your way into the senatorial and equestrian class, but it was your behaviour that made you one of the *infames*. This could be linked to sexual transgressions: women successfully prosecuted for adultery would be classed *infames*, as would men who had consented to penetration by another man. Or for other circumstances that were considered lacking in honour, such as bankruptcy, dishonourable discharge from the army or being convicted of a (non-sexual) criminal charge.

The easiest way to acquire *infamia* status was by your profession for it was an unavoidable consequence of certain occupations. The most notable of these tainted professionals were some of the most famous people in Rome, gladiators. Also included in this group were actors, pimps and prostitutes.

Those who had acquired *infamia* could not speak on behalf of others in a court of law, they could not bring accusations against others, they couldn't vote, they were barred from participating in government and they couldn't serve in the army. Without citizenship they were liable to public beatings or corporal punishment. And as noted, they were forbidden from marrying any free person. It was no small deal to be classed as an *infamis*.

Prostitution

As well as the legal restrictions placed on the *infames* as described above, prostitutes had an added condition placed upon them: they were forbidden from wearing the *stola* of the respectable Roman woman. Instead they wore togas, a visual demonstration of their lack of honour and *virtus*.

Despite all these rules dedicated to singling out and isolating prostitutes from respectable Romans of all classes, prostitution was legal and even taxable. The canny Caligula had spotted an opportunity for profit and introduced a tax on each trick performed, although how this was calculated and collected is anyone's guess.

Suetonius, our biographer of the Caesars, also wrote a work entitled *On Famous Prostitutes*. The title itself is intriguing and suggests that some prostitutes could obtain fame and notoriety, perhaps equivalent to their fellow *infames*, actresses. Sadly, we will never know the names of these famous prostitutes since Suetonius' work has been lost, but that it ever existed as a book at all tells us something of the nature of ancient prostitution; it was varied.

At the very high end would have been the concubine, the likely subjects of Suetonius' lost work. There are a few names that we can pluck out of history, most notably in the Republican era, for example Flora who was courtesan to Pompey the Great. It was a triumph she never forgot and when in her old age would tell stories about that time: '[She] always took delight in telling about her former intimacy with Pompey, saying that she never left his embraces without bearing the marks of his teeth.'[8]

Pompey appears to be not so enamoured of Flora, for when his friend Geminius expressed an interest in her, Pompey handed her over to him, a situation that left Flora sick with grief and longing. Pompey not so much. In fact, not at all.

A courtesan who achieved higher influence than Flora was Praecia, who Plutarch tells us was famed for her wit and beauty, but also for her connections. 'In other respects she was no whit better than an ordinary courtesan, but she used her associates and companions to further the political ambitions of her friends, and so added to her other charms the reputation of being a true comrade, and one who could bring things to pass.'[9]

One of her biggest conquests was the Roman politician Publius Cornelius Cethegus who came to depend on her so completely that he undertook no public measure unless she had approved it. Such was her influence that it is the general Lucullus who has to court her with gifts and flattery. Lucullus' desire for Praecia was purely transactional: he wanted something from her that was not sex related – an introduction to her lover, Cethegus. This he gets and the influential Cethegus helps him secure a provincial governorship.

The story of Praecia is not dissimilar to those Republican era marriages contracted to bind families together to the mutual benefit of each other. Courting Praecia gains Lucullus access to Cethegus, Praecia gains kudos from being seen with Lucullus, which may benefit her financially as others try to buy her influence, and Cethegus gets an introduction to rising star Lucullus that might do him some good in the future. Everyone is happy. At least until Lucullus, having got what he wanted, has no further use for Praecia and Cethegus and ditches the pair of them. We might speculate that Lucullus didn't want to tarnish his *virtus* by consorting with a famous prostitute or we might just conclude that he was mercenary.

Elsewhere at the highest levels of society the emperors were getting involved in the oldest profession. Caligula, Suetonius tells us, set up a grand brothel in the palace itself with the added twist that the prostitutes working in this brothel were matrons and freeborn boys. As both these groups are covered under the Lex Scantinia, what Caligula is offering to his punters is a chance to taste forbidden fruit and enjoy the illicit pleasure of breaking a taboo.

Tacitus has a similar tale when recounting a party that the head of the Praetorian Guard, Tigellinus, threw for Nero. Included amongst the entertainment were a series of brothels set up by a lakeside, all staffed by freeborn women of high rank. If that failed to please the boss, Tigellinus had a whole heap of naked harlots of very low rank on standby.

Outside of these imperial endeavours there is mention of prostitution at work within the palace. Nymphidia Sabina was the mother of the Praetorian Prefect, Nymphidius Sabinus, who persuaded the guard to abandon Nero, thus pushing the emperor into his flight from Rome and suicide. She gets but a couple of lines in the recorded history, but they are belters. Tacitus describes her as having prostituted herself amongst the slaves and freedmen of the palace. But she went beyond the staff for she was said to have also slept with Caligula, who Tacitus dryly notes had an appetite for a harlot. Her son would later claim he was the son of Caligula, but he wasn't, the most likely candidate was a gladiator named Martianus.

Nymphidia was evidently well known since Plutarch puts a speech in the mouth of the Praetorian Guard Antonius Honoratus where he questions whether they should be 'choosing the son of Nymphidia as our Caesar.'[10] Note that it is enough to just say her name, he doesn't need to spell out her profession. Here perhaps is a famous whore at last.

If an emperor was stepping into the high-end brothel business, we might assume that others were too, but finding evidence of this is not easy. In fact, finding evidence of the existence of any kind of brothel is fraught with difficulty.[11] How do we identify a particular building as a brothel?

As we've discussed in previous chapters, Romans were a crude lot given to recording their crudity on the sides of buildings, so should we take graffiti such as 'I screwed a lot of girls here' as proof that the building was a brothel? Similarly, should we consider a building with a lot of explicit erotic images as a brothel? That would mean that Pompeii was a town with a brothel for pretty much every citizen and their slave. And did those penises carved onto the flagstones really point the way to a brothel, or were they simply there as good luck symbols? Calculating the number of brothels in a town that has miraculously survived nearly intact from two millennia ago is not as simple as you might suppose.

The latest research estimates that Pompeii had thirty-five brothels, which works out as one brothel for every seventy-five free adult males. Not included in these calculations, because we have no way of ascertaining their numbers, are those visiting Pompeii on business or pleasure, or deciding to combine the two with a brothel trip.

One example of a brothel in Pompeii stands behind the town bath house, the Lupanar. This is a grim building; its ground floor is divided into five narrow, cell-like rooms. In these rooms, taking up all the space, are stone beds on which, presumably, softer mattresses and pillows would have been placed. There are no windows in any of the cells, nor have any doors been found. The assumption is that maybe all that divided them from view was a curtain, or perhaps not even that. Upstairs are five more rooms, slightly wider than the floor below but again with stone beds.

Within the brothel there have been found over 100 examples of graffiti, all of it is of an explicit nature. Included in these wall scribblings are the prices charged by the individual girls and what services you might purchase, for example, 'Euplia sucks for five asses.' Also reviews from happy or unhappy punters, 'Sollemnes, you screw well!', and the sort of general bawdiness you would probably expect from a house selling sex.

Erotic paintings adorn this building, with the most famous showing couples engaged in a variety of sexual positions, leaving some scholars to wonder whether this was a menu of a sort. Did you look at these pictures and then chose the sexual position you wanted? It's a neat idea but we have no clue whether there is any truth in it.

Was there a stigma about visiting a brothel? Artemidorus, our dream interpreter extraordinaire, suggests there was: 'To have sex with prostitutes based in brothels signifies a little bit of shame and some small expense, as men who consort with these girls are both ashamed and out of pocket.'[12]

The men who visited a brothel were likely to be of a low class. The wealthy did not tend to frequent brothels because they did not need to, they could afford to buy slaves to satisfy their every sexual whim. Which makes you wonder whether there ever was such a thing as a high-class brothel for the discerning rich man. The examples on offer in Pompeii, a rich prosperous town, would suggest not.

Brothels were not the only place to buy sex, there appears to have been quite a trade going on in bars. A great number of the graffiti found in Pompeii and Herculaneum involves boasts about screwing barmaids. Clearly there was some skulduggery afoot to escape the prostitute tax by claiming that the barmaids are just that, serving drinks and nothing more. The law, though, is having none of it: 'If anyone running a tavern has women for hire (and many are accustomed to have female prostitutes under the guise of having tavern maids) then she is properly called a madam.'[13]

There's a dry joke in an inscription found at Aesernia, where an innkeeper hands over the bill to her guest. He is charged one ass for bread and wine, one ass for meat, two asses for hay for his mule and two asses for sex with the barmaid. That mule will be the end of me, the guest retorts.

At the very much lower end of the scale were the street walkers. We get the word fornication from *fornices* meaning arches, which is where prostitutes would tout for business. As the defining feature of pretty much all Roman public buildings, arches gave a lot of scope for encounters. The fact that street walkers were at the bottom of the heap is shown by this Martial poem:

I want an easy mantle-wearing girl, who strolls around
I want one who has already given herself to my slave;
I want one who sells her whole self for a denarius or two ...'[14]

Obviously, the more people the more scope there was for a prostitute to make money. Outside the theatre, the circus and the amphitheatre were key areas for sex workers, who no doubt hoped the 'performances' had stirred the lust of the spectators. If they'd attended the theatre, they might well have seen themselves portrayed, for the prostitute was a stock character in comedy plays.

The comic plays of Plautus have a recurring theme: a young man falls in love with a beautiful prostitute and desires to have her to himself. A series of misadventures then occur as the young man, with the help of his clever slave, tries to get the money together to buy his girl. At the end it is revealed that the prostitute is not a prostitute at all but a freeborn girl. This counts as a happy ending since the young man can now marry the girl.

This plotline features in his play *Poenulus* in which the prostitute character has been kidnapped as a baby from Carthage and is reunited with her father who reveals her freeborn status. It's used in *Curculio*, where the young prostitute runs into her brother who reveals her freeborn status, thus allowing her to wed her young man. It's again used in *Pseudolus*, but though the prostitute Phoenicium is not revealed at the end to be freeborn, she still gets a happy ending with her admiring young man.

It is interesting that part of these stock plots involve a freeborn girl being kidnapped and sold into slavery/prostitution. Was this a real fear of the Romans that Plautus is reflecting? Loss of freedom, status and citizen rights was certainly every Roman's nightmare given the highly class-based, judgmental society they lived in and the rights that citizenship gave.

There is evidence that the freeborn, despite protection under the law, could be sold into slavery. In 69 CE, during the civil war between Otho and Vitellius, the town of Cremona was sacked, and, to the horror of Tacitus, freeborn citizens of Rome were captured by the soldiers and sold as slaves.

The second thing we may gauge from Plautus is something on the restrictive nature of Roman courting. As we've previously explored, marriage was an arranged contract between families, and freeborn women's virtue was protected. Therefore, Plautus' tales of young men falling for prostitutes is the socially acceptable love story – prostitutes don't have *stuprum* allowing them to be courted and loved by the young man. Significantly, the prostitute is shown to be free at the end of the tale, and so, unknowing, she cannot be held responsible for any behaviour earlier in the play that would be unseemly for the freeborn.

Actors and actresses

There were different types of actors and acting in Rome: dancers and mime artists, comic actors and those giving their all in Greek tragedy. Although the type of role they performed had no impact on their status, the acting profession as a whole was labelled *infamia*, the tragic actor in the serious play was as damned as the performer in a crude, bawdy mime.

In the marriage laws not only were the higher classes banned from marrying actors or actresses but also the sons and daughters of actors. Actors were considered highly dubious, as the proclamation below from the third century shows. Note that although the charioteer gets no comment, the actor is 'vile': 'If the portrait of a buffoon in short garments, or one of a charioteer with wrinkled breast, or of a vile actor, should be placed in the public porticoes, or anywhere in the city in which our statues are usually erected, it shall immediately be removed; nor shall it, hereafter, ever be lawful for the representations of such degraded persons to be exhibited in respectable places.'[15]

The proclamation concludes with an allowance that statues of these 'degraded persons' can be placed in the porticos of the theatre, their proper place. Juvenal sees the theatre as invoking female lusts, 'They'll pay a fortune to get an actor's clasp undone,'[16] he dryly says. Ovid recommends the theatre as a good place to pick up women, 'this place is fatal to chastity.'

Mark Antony's general debauched reputation included dalliances with the acting profession. He was a friend to several mime actors to the degree that he even attended their weddings. During one such nuptial he took full advantage of the free bar and kept the drinking up all night long, which didn't turn out so well when he was summoned to the Forum on official business and threw up all over his toga.

Vomiting during sacred public duties aside, Antony's most famous dalliance with the acting profession was an affair with the actress, Cytheris. She accompanied Antony in his litter on his city visits and, as Plutarch tells us, she had as many attendants bestowed upon her as Antony had given his mother. Which is something that annoys Cicero no end, 'Antony, for his part, is carrying about Cytheris with him with his sedan open, as a second wife,'[17] adding, 'See what disgraceful circumstances we are being done to death!'

He refers to Antony disparagingly as 'that lover of Cytheris', which had to be awkward when he later found himself at the same dinner party as her: 'To tell you the truth, I had no suspicion that she would be there.'[18] Still he mans up, explaining to his correspondent that 'the fact is that that sort of thing never had any attraction for me when I was a young man, much less now I am an old one.' As if Cytheris is going to throw herself at Cicero! Cytheris' crime is to act as a respectable woman might, attending dinner parties and travelling with Antony on official business. She has got above herself and her place in the class system.

Actors were clearly very sexy, because not only did they drive the girls at the theatre crazy with lust, they could similarly attract the highest-ranked lovers in the land. Caligula was very much taken by a pantomime actor by the name of Mnester, 'If anyone made even the slightest sound while his favourite was dancing, he had him dragged from his seat and scourged him with his own hand.'[19]

Like Antony before him, Caligula took his lust too far and was seen to kiss Mnester in public, as Suetonius notes: 'Toward those to whom he was devoted his partiality became madness.'[20]

After Caligula's assassination there was a vote to melt down all coins that contained his image. The Empress Messalina, wife of new the new emperor, Claudius, asked if she could make use of this metal. She made use of it by having a bronze statue of Mnester cast, which was the initial hint that Messalina might quite fancy the actor. Later she compelled him to be her lover, a move that proved unpopular with the public, who also adored Mnester and were fed up that he was no longer performing for them (because he was busy performing in another fashion for Messalina).

Other actors who attracted an imperial eye include Paris, who enjoyed a liaison with Domitian's wife, Domitia, at least until Domitian had him murdered. Martial writes a rather touching epithet for him, 'Whoever you are, traveller, that tread the Flaminian way, pass not unheeded this noble tomb. The delight of the city, the wit of the Nile, the art and grace, the sportiveness and joy, the glory and grief of the Roman theatre, and all its Venuses and Cupids, lie buried in this tomb, with Paris.'[21]

Evidently Paris, like Mnester before him, was a hugely popular actor with the public, although not to be confused with another Paris who was also an actor but this time in Nero's reign (Nero had that Paris killed because he would not teach him mime).

Whereas prostitution existed within Roman society quite happily and without much commentary in our sources, the same cannot be said for actors and the theatre. They were troublesome.

Aside from causing marital discord within the imperial household, actors were also causing discord on the streets of Rome. Remember that quote about Caligula's partiality turning to madness in relation to his favourite actor, Mnester? Caligula was far from alone in that sentiment. Actors attracted devoted followers who formed themselves into factions determined to protect the reputation and honour of their beloved. You can probably guess what's coming: yep, there were street battles between factions, not unlike the football hooligans of old.

Such was the violence that stern measures were taken. Under the Emperor Tiberius several actors found themselves banished from Rome along with their fans. 'When a quarrel in the theatre ended in bloodshed, he banished the leaders of the factions, as well as the actors who were the cause of the dissension; and no entreaties of the people could ever induce him to recall them.'[22]

Tacitus fills in a few more details about this incident. Apparently several soldiers and a centurion were killed in the riot and a member of the Praetorian Guard injured while trying to restore order. This was not an isolated incident; we get a similar tale of riots and expulsions from Rome during Nero's reign, although this time it's the pantomime actors getting into a fight. Suetonius tells us that Nero himself used to go to the theatre to egg on the fighting actors and that, 'When they came to blows and fought with stones and broken benches, he himself threw many missiles at the people and even broke a praetor's head.'[23]

We do not get stories along these lines relating to prostitution. Actors were dangerously sexy, so dangerously sexy that they inspired extreme violence. Is it any wonder that the Romans considered them *infames*?

Gladiators

Gladiators were classed as *infames* and their ranks were predominantly filled by slaves. It was possible to volunteer as a gladiator, which involved forfeiting your rights to protection under the law for a set period of time or a certain number of bouts, but we have no way of knowing how many men did this. Most inscriptions to gladiators show them to have been slaves.

Gladiators are a peculiar mix, categorised as the lowest of the low in society they nonetheless possessed the epic courage and skill in fighting that was classed as *virtus*. It was a difficult conundrum for the Romans: were these people worthy of fraternising with or were they as lacking in reputation and honour as all *infames* were? It wasn't something that was easily resolved, and gladiators occupy a strange position in society.

Gladiators were sufficiently famous as to be a merchandisable commodity, appearing on oil lamps and glass wear. The over-the-top freedman in Petronius' *Satyricon*, Trimalcho, is the proud owner of some gladiator merchandise of his own: 'And I have got the fights between Hereros and Petraites on my cups, and every cup is a heavy one; for I do not sell my connoisseurship for any money.'[24]

They are the subject of adulation from the people, as demonstrated by this graffiti found on the gladiator barracks in Pompeii, 'Celadus the Thracian gladiator. Girls think he's magnificent!' That these girls are unnamed, and given where the graffiti was found, does make you wonder whether Celadus himself is the author of this sentiment. Perhaps it is an attempt to raise his profile?

Given that gladiators fought in the semi-nude with their muscles on full display it is not surprising that they garnered an appreciative female following. Juvenal has the story of Eppia who deserted her senator husband and children to run away with the gladiator, Sergius. Sergius, Juvenal maintains, was not even that handsome; 'His face was seriously disfigured, a furrow chafed by his helmet, a huge lump on the bridge of his nose, And a nasty condition provoking a forever-weeping eye.'[25]

But, as Juvenal concludes, he was a gladiator and that gave him an allure, a sex appeal despite his appearance. What is surprising, given the gladiator's noted sex appeal and allure, is that there are not similar accounts to that of Eppia. Whereas actors find themselves the lovers of emperors, empresses and other notable elites, we just don't get the same kind of stories about gladiators. There is no Paris, Cytheris or Mnester of the gladiatorial world.

It is true that in the gladiator barracks in Pompeii there was found the body of a richly dressed woman. This has garnered lots of speculation that she was there for a bit of nude fraternisation with the gods of the arena. Alternatively, and more likely, she'd gone there to shelter when the raining ash became too heavy for her to continue her journey.

The nearest we get is a suggestion that Faustina, the wife of Marcus Aurelius, may have had an affair with a gladiator. This is used to explain how the great Marcus Aurelius managed to produce such a useless gladiator-obsessed son, Commodus. In one version of the story Faustina doesn't even have sex with the gladiator but rather forms a strong passion for him. After immediately confessing all to her husband, the emperor consults resident magicians who advise that the empress bathe in the blood of this gladiator and then have sex with her husband. There are no details given on how much blood Faustina was ordered to put in her bath or whether the gladiator in question survived this bloodletting. In fact, gladiator blood was a potent mix, so potent that it was used as an ingredient for love potions, epilepsy and infertility.

It's worth noting that the thing that all three professions have in common is public performance, something that caused a shiver of horror down the spine of any good Roman. So shameful was performing in public that the stain could last generations. 'They are dead and I feel I owe it to their ancestors not to name them,'[26] says Tacitus of the equestrian men who took part in Nero's performances. He has stronger words for the emperor himself: deplorable, degrading, corrupted, disgrace. That Nero enjoyed playing the lyre, driving chariots and writing poetry was not the crime, doing so in public was.

Given that Romans happily went to the toilet together in communal latrines, bathed naked together in the public baths and routinely had sex in front of their slaves without thinking about it, this distaste is not connected with any concept of privacy. It seems rather to be linked to giving pleasure to others (which is where prostitutes fit in) with an added shame level of doing so in public that is so abhorrent to the Roman mind.

Incest

There were places in the ancient world where incest was ingrained at the highest level. Ancient Egypt is perhaps the best-known example where it became customary for the ruling Pharaoh to marry his sister. Cleopatra, for instance, clocked up two marriages to two of her brothers.

In Rome the pantheon of gods were old hands at incest: Jupiter, the king of the Gods, was married to his sister Juno, and had a daughter, Proserpina, by his sister Ceres. Proserpina is later abducted and marries her own uncle, Pluto. Ceres has another daughter by her brother Neptune. I could go on, and on.

Unlike other religions, the Roman gods were not there as examples to emulate, or even be inspired by. They lived extreme lives of violence, sex, bestiality and adultery on an epic scale that no sane person would wish to follow (or be able to keep up with). The gods were to be feared, placated and buttered up with sacrifices and offerings.

Sex with children may have been culturally tolerated, even celebrated (under certain conditions), but incest was most definitely not. I say this with confidence because it pops up as a slur in those barbed speeches that Roman politicians lob at each other with the ferocity of a slingshot.

Cicero, the master at these no-holds-barred, reputation-stripping invectives, uses incest to damn his rivals. Most notably Publius Clodius, who he repeatedly accuses of incest with his sister, Clodia, sometimes with a nod and a wink, 'I had not a quarrel with that woman's husband – brother, I meant to say; I am always making this mistake.'[27] Insert knowing chuckle of laughter from the spectators.

Sometimes far more blatantly, such as in a speech attacking Clodia when he brings up her illustrious ancestors and what they might think of her behaviour: 'Was it for this that I brought water to Rome, for you to bathe in it after your incestuous couplings?'[28]

As a prominent politician of his age, it is unsurprising to find the same accusation flung straight back at Cicero. 'This man who has shown so great licentiousness and impurity throughout his entire life that he would not spare even his closest kin but let out his wife for hire and was his daughter's lover.'[29]

Accusations of incest against emperors appear too frequently in our sources to remain wholly, or even slightly credible. They read very much like another entry on the agreed checklist of what makes an emperor depraved. Think of any emperor with a reputation for excess and I can pretty much guarantee they are also accused of incest.

Caligula? Slept with all three of his sisters. Nero? Slept with his mother. Domitian? Affair with his niece. Commodus? Sisters again. Caracalla? Ditto with the mother love.

Aside from damning an emperor as distinctly lacking in *virtus* and being an out and out pervert, there is lurking behind some of these incest allegations a large dollop of misogyny. Nowhere is this more apparent than in the tale of Agrippina.

Family machinations – Agrippina the younger

Agrippina was one of those imperial ladies who is connected to everyone. She was the granddaughter of Julia, the daughter of Augustus, the niece of Claudius and the sister of Caligula. She had survived Sejanus' machinations, she had survived exile by her brother, she had survived Messalina's petty vindictiveness and now she was determined that her son would be emperor.

This determination is quite something to witness; there was little that Agrippina wasn't prepared to do to drape her son in purple. Whether he was worth her efforts is open to debate, and certainly she questioned it herself later.

Her first step was to get her son married to the Emperor Claudius' daughter, Octavia. Octavia was already betrothed to someone else, but this was no impediment to Agrippina. Strange and unpleasant rumours surfaced about Octavia's fiancé, Torquatus, linking him to an unnatural relationship with his sister. These rumours spread far enough to give Claudius second thoughts about marrying him to his daughter and the betrothal was broken off. Step one accomplished.

Now that her son was successfully betrothed to an emperor's daughter, Agrippina embarked on step two of her make-my son-emperor masterplan, i.e., become empress. Handily, the previous empress, Messalina, had been recently decapitated for illicit shenanigans of the highest order, which had left an opening for Agrippina. There was just one problem, Claudius happened to be her uncle and any relationship between them would therefore be considered incest and illegal.

But nay, what is the moral and legal code of society to a woman of these ambitions? It is but a twig to be snapped out of the way. Besides, one of the perks of being emperor is that you can get those pesky laws that get in your way changed. Which is exactly what Claudius did and only a day later married Agrippina.

Aside from ultimate wealth and power, Claudius didn't have much going for him: 'He would foam at the mouth and trickle at the nose; he stammered besides and his head was very shaky at all times, but especially when he made the least exertion.'[30]

Which might explain step three on Agrippina's plan: murder her husband. Claudius was poisoned by a dish of mushrooms, of all things. Agrippina had clearly used those seductive powers throughout their marriage, for Claudius made her son, Nero, emperor rather than his own son, Britannicus.

What with seducing your less-than-attractive uncle, engaging in political rumour-mongering and wholesale murder solely on behalf of your son, you might expect him to be a tad grateful. But teenage boys are not known for their regard towards their mothers. Was it any wonder that Agrippina was infuriated when Nero was suddenly spending all his time with his mistress, the imperial freedwoman Acte? She was losing her grip on her son and once she had lost that, with it went her influence.

Her response, according to our sources, was somewhat extreme; she set to seducing her son, offering up her bedroom for private activities. Suetonius, naturally, has the raciest account, 'Whenever he rode in a litter with his mother, he had incestuous relations with her, which were betrayed by the stains on his clothing.' Yuck.

It is worth noting that the bit before that Suetonius quote is, 'so they say'. So *they* say; 'they' being anonymous. There are no witnesses to this incest named anywhere. It is handily said to happen in closed litters and behind closed doors, from which I think we can conclude that it is absolute rubbish.

Rubbish it may be, but it tells us something about how Agrippina and other powerful women were viewed. Women could not hold public offices or vote, and were entirely excluded from politics. The assumption of the Roman man, therefore, is that they only have one thing they can use to influence events, their bodies. The fact that Agrippina was an extremely clever woman doesn't enter their thought processes; sex was her power

---

firstly with her brother, Caligula, then her uncle, Claudius, then her son, Nero. How else could she have risen to such a position of influence? Agrippina certainly used sex. A later affair with the influential freedman Pallas no doubt aided her survival during a period of fierce competition amongst palace freedmen, but she had a lot more going for her than that.

There is a question about incest we haven't touched upon yet and which needs asking. We've discussed in a previous chapter just how much intermarriage there was in the ruling dynasties of Rome: the Julio Claudians particularly become horribly intermeshed marriage-wise. For example, when Tiberius married Augustus' daughter, Julia, he was marrying both his stepsister and his former mother-in-law. His brother Drusus got off relatively lightly in comparison by marrying only his step-cousin. Let's ask the question, what counted as incest?

That Claudius made marriage between uncles and nieces legal did not suddenly make it a fashion. There remained a distaste to such liaisons, as shown by how the Claudius/Agrippina marriage is depicted. A similar distaste is evident in accounts of Domitian's alleged affair with his niece, Julia, though this was not illegal nor counted as incest. Juvenal is particularly damning of him, 'Domitian, that recent adulterer, behaved, defiled by a fatal union,' adding in this vile image, 'While Julia, his niece, ditched the contents of her ripe womb with abortifacients, and shed lumps resembling her uncle.'[31]

The law that Claudius introduced was very specific. Agrippina was the daughter of Claudius' brother, Germanicus, but any marriage between a man and his sister's children was still deemed as incest. Also, a woman could not marry her nephew, whether he was the son of her sister or her brother. This strange double standard, which seems only to come about solely because Claudius wanted to marry Agrippina, was finally resolved in the fourth century when joint emperors Constans and Constanius made marriage between a man and his niece, whether she be his brother's or sister's child, one of the many offences punishable by death during that era.

Paulus, a third-century jurist, states that incest is counted when a man marries a woman who is either a descendant or an ascendent of his, which would have excluded pretty much all the marriages of the Julio Claudian dynasty.

Most of the laws regarding incest are concerned with inheritance rights and dowries: 'Incestuous marriages confer no right of dowry, and therefore the husband can be deprived of everything which he receives, even though it comes under the head of profits.'[32]

The concentration on incest in ancient Rome is all to do with legality or illegality, there is little in the way of recognition that incest might be sexual abuse, as we would think of it today. There is, however, this rather unsettling legal pronouncement: 'If adultery is committed at the same time as incest, for instance, with a stepdaughter, a daughter-in-law, or a stepmother, the woman shall also be punished, for this will take place even where adultery was not committed.'[33]

This does conjure up horrific images of a stepdaughter being abused and then facing prosecution for the abuse perpetrated by her stepfather upon her, but this doesn't seem to figure in the ancient Roman mind. The laws on incest are concerned with inheritance rights and what happens when someone unknowingly makes an incestuous marriage. Unknowingly entering into an incestuous marriage was apparently an often-enough circumstance to need spelling out in law. However, there is leniency in these accounts, and women are let off incest charges due to their age or ignorance of the law. The caveat being this is incest committed via illegal marriages, otherwise parties would also fall foul under the adultery legislation.

Does this mean that interfamilial abuse did not feature in ancient Rome? It certainly features in some of the dreams that Artemidorus collected: there are sections for dreams about penetrating a daughter and penetrating a son that appear under a larger heading of 'Intercourse contrary to nature.' Artemidorus is very clear how wrong this act was, 'no one in his right mind would penetrate anyone at that age, let alone his son.'[34] The age in question here is under five years old. That it features again and again in political slurs show how taboo and contrary to nature, as Artemidorus puts it, incest was felt to be by Romans.

Bestiality

Designated as the most contrary to nature by Artemidorus, bestiality, like incest, features heavily in the stories of the gods. Jupiter kidnapped Europa in the guise of a bull and impregnated Leda while being a swan.

The minotaur was the product of a union between Queen Paisphae and a bull she had taken a fancy to. The act itself was achieved by Paisphae hiding within a specially built wooden cow and waiting until the object of her affection mounted the sexy fake cow, the queen making sure she was in the correct position.

Bestiality also featured in art, including an impressive statue of Pan having it away with a goat. This was locked away in the Museum of Naples' secret cabinet because it was just too good (and which we will discuss in a later chapter). The story of Leda and the swan was a particular favourite with Pompeii householders, including one newly discovered fresco. Oil lamps also featured depictions of man versus beast in unnatural couplings including dogs, ponies and donkeys.

In literature Apuleius, who we last saw successfully denying he was a magician, wrote a novel called *The Golden Ass* which features, as you're no doubt expecting now, sex between woman and ass. A disturbingly sexy scene includes the ass (who is really our hero Lucius who has been turned into the creature by a witch) worrying about the damage he might inflict upon his partner, 'But I was greatly troubled by no small fear, thinking in what manner should I be able, with legs so many and of such a size, to mount a tender and highborn lady – in what manner my gentlewoman could support so gigantic a genital?'35

Juvenal alleges that so highly sexed are women that they are not averse to anal sex with animals, 'And there's a lack of men, not a moment slips by, before she'll accommodate her arse, freely, to a donkey's rude attentions.'36

By which point I think we are all probably behind Artemidorus in classing all of the above as sexual intercourse contrary to nature. The question, though, demands to be asked: what is wrong with these people? Was bestiality really a bit of titillation in ancient Rome, something to add to your interior décor and throw in as a side plot in your comic novel?

We've discussed previously that the actions of the gods were certainly not something that was to be emulated, but they were stories that were to be represented in art, bestiality included. There is something in both Juvenal and Apuleius' accounts that is playing to stereotypes of the oversexed and insatiable woman, so we might consider that as satire rather than a depiction of reality.

But there is one account of bestiality that is not so easy to shake off as a joke and it comes from a series of poems by Martial on the games.

The games had a set programme: the morning was given over to beast hunts and the afternoon to gladiator combats. Squeezed in-between these two highly popular entertainments was the execution of criminals, which took place at around noon.

Because Rome had no working police force or criminal justice system in the way we would recognise, punishments had to be public to put off all those would-be offenders. They also had to be bloody and painful as a further deterrent. What they weren't, however, was terribly entertaining, something that Seneca complains about in a letter: 'It is pure murder. The men have no protective covering. Their entire bodies are exposed to the blows, and no blow is ever struck in vain [...] In the morning men are thrown to the lions and the bears, at noon they are thrown to their spectators.'[37]

As a way of making this essential bit of social machinery more palatable the criminals were dressed up and forced to partake in a restaging of a famous myth, one during which they would obviously meet their state-approved death. Martial mentions several of these mythological re-enactments. There is one recounting Prometheus having his liver pecked out by a vulture, except they clearly couldn't get a vulture, or the vulture was uncooperative, for it is substituted for a bear which rips out the entrails of the criminal for the crowd's pleasure. Another staging was that of Daedulus who flew too close to the sun, melting the wax on his wings and plummeting to his death, or in this example into the path of another bear.

'While you were being thus torn by a Lucanian bear, how must you have desired to have those wings of yours,' comments an entirely unsympathetic Martial. Which brings us to the next re-enactment about which Martial writes a poem. It's a story we encountered earlier, that of Paisphae and the bull:

> Pasiphae really was mated to that Cretan bull:
> believe it: we've seen it, the old story's true.
> old antiquity needn't pride itself so, Caesar:
> whatever legend sings, the arena offers you.[38]

This raises a very unpleasant question: did the Romans really execute female criminals by way of being raped by a bull? Martial offers us nothing more on the subject and there are no other references to such an act in the arena. But this part of the games gets scant attention in any case, being overshadowed by those exciting beast hunts and glamorous gladiators.

If we think back to Nero's favourite eunuch, Sporus, he committed suicide rather than appear in a production of the rape of Proserpina. Vitellius was intending to portray the rape at the heart of the story for real, which might suggest that the Paisphae story was also enacted for real. The truth is we simply can't know for sure, but it leaves a very unpleasant taste in the mouth.

Chapter 15

Sexual Imagery

Upstairs in the British Museum there is a room dedicated to the Roman Empire. It is filled with all the artefacts you'd expect to see: coins aplenty, amphora, busts of emperors long gone and a really quite terrifying head of Augustus.[1] But there's something else that is important enough to get a glass case of its own, a certain silver drinking vessel (see image 26).

You approach the case, intrigued by the polished silver. Staring through the glass, you begin to take in the picture expertly carved into the cup and realise you are examining a scene that shows a young man lowering himself onto the erect penis of an older, bearded man. This is the point where you either step back blushing or immediately head down to the gift shop to buy a replica. It can go either way.

The Warren Cup, as this silver vessel is known, dates to the Augustan period. Its provenance is somewhat murky. The British Museum say it may have come from the Levant, adding in a 'probably'. The cup was 'said to have been found' near Jerusalem and was 'likely' commissioned by a member of the Greek community of the Eastern Mediterranean. All of which is curator speak for a shrug of the shoulders.

The Warren Cup is not a singular object but one of many on the same theme. Although its exquisite carving and silver material elevate it above others in the genre, depictions of men having sex features on cups, cameos rings and most other types of crockery.

The Warren Cup was an expensive bit of such crockery, and its owner, whoever that may have been, was unlikely to have hidden it away. This was a cup to show off, as indeed the British Museum is doing to this day.

A large range of said objects have been found during the excavations of Pompeii and Herculaneum, to the disillusionment of the excavators. Was the culture that produced the likes of Cicero, Augustus and Scipio really the same culture that apparently owned a statue of the god Pan having it away with a goat? Not to mention the terracotta penises that filled box after box.

Then there were the frescos that decorated the walls of well-to-do homes, frescos that were deemed so shocking that the excavators chipped them off the walls and hurried with their wheelbarrows of pottery penises to a secret room in Naples where they would spend their days.

The so-called secret cabinet in Naples museum was the receptacle of these graphic objects that the archaeologists struggled to explain. It's still a struggle today. We think we know what all those carved phalluses were for but it's still a bit of guesswork.

What the excavations of Pompeii revealed was a culture that was bombarded by what we would call sexual or even erotic images. You could be drinking out of a cup displaying anal sex, have a fresco on your wall of a man and woman going for it and hang a carved penis outside your house. You might then stroll to the nearest wall and scrawl on it how you really like oral sex, just in case anyone wants to know. It's a very perplexing world. Is it any wonder the archaeologists lobbed everything in a cabinet, turned the key and told each other they'd work it all out later?

What was your average resident of Pompeii thinking when he invited in the decorators and told them to paint a whopping great image of a woman having sex with a swan? Grand Designs this certainly isn't. Why are there so many penises everywhere, from carvings in the pavement and masonry to necklaces and rings, and pottery ones for the home? Who owned that magnificent statue of Pan and the goat, and why did he buy it? And why was anal sex a suitable subject for your favourite mug?

There is a lot to unpick here. In book ten of his *Metamorphoses*, Ovid recounts the story of Pygmalion, the sculptor who fell in love with a statue he had crafted himself. In Ovid's hands this tale is less the plot of the movie *Mannequin* and more about a creepy loner who gets his kicks tickling the ivory because he's been turned off the fairer sex. 'He arranges the statue on a bed on which cloths dyed with Tyrian murex are spread, and calls it his bedfellow, and rests its neck against soft down, as if it could feel,' breathes Ovid. 'He kisses it and thinks his kisses are returned; and speaks to it; and holds it and imagines that his fingers press into the limbs.'

Pygmalion, having presumably spent some time playing with his ivory mistress, attends the local festival for the goddess Venus. Standing at the altar having made his sacrifice, he asks the goddess for a bride just like his statue. Venus grants him his wish and turns his ivory statue into a real girl.

Pliny the Elder has the tale of another alluring statue, this time one of the goddess Venus herself, carved by the famous sculptor Praxiteles. Pliny tells us how fabulous a statue it was, 'it is admirable from every angle!' he marvels, before telling us, 'There is a story that a man who had fallen in love with the statue hid in the temple at night and embraced it intimately; a stain bears witness to his lust.'[2]

I bring up these two stories because we are going to talk about that fact that what we see as erotically charged scenes, explicit pornography even, is not what the Romans saw. Though, as these two stories show, sometimes they most certainly did.

'Surely in your house, just as figures of great men of old shrine – painted by some artists' hand – so somewhere a small picture depicts the various forms of copulations and sexual positions.' Here, Ovid, in exile,[3] addresses the Emperor Augustus, of all people. 'Surely' he says not as a question but as a statement. The poet is not prepared to believe that even the morality machine Augustus does not have these pictures in his house. The underlying meaning is clear: everybody does.

One person we can say with certainty who did have such images is Augustus' own stepson and successor, Tiberius. Suetonius tells us he collected the most salacious of paintings and sculptures, as well as setting up an 'erotic library'. Which I'm presuming means it was filled with books of erotica, rather than it being a particularly sexy place to hang out.

In 53 BCE the Parthians were shocked to find a collection of erotic stories in the baggage of the Roman soldiers they had just comprehensively annihilated in an ambush. They were amazed that, even when marching into war, the Romans could not be parted from their sex books.

Interestingly, one of Soranus' suggestions for women suffering from what might be gonorrhoea is not to show them paintings of shapely forms or tell them erotic stories. That this advice had to be written down is suggestive that looking at arousing pictures and telling sexy stories was a familiar and acceptable pastime.

The evidence found in Pompeii and Herculaneum certainly backs up Ovid's confidence that everybody has pictures of copulation and sexual positions in their house. The House of the Vettii, for instance, has a fresco depicting a couple in the missionary position and another showing a woman being taken from behind by a man. The House of Caecilus has a fresco of woman on top of a man, but this time facing away from her partner. The House of the Centenary has a similar depiction of a woman squatting on a man's penis, facing away from him. And we could keep going.

These are all private houses, so were these erotic frescoes for the owner's private enjoyment, much like the Emperor Tiberius and his erotic collection? The answer to this question could lie in the location of these frescoes within the house. If they were in a bedroom, for instance, we might conclude they were a private fantasy builder for the house owner to whip up his libido pre-quiet night in with the wife (or other chosen partner). If they were in a dining room, less so.

The homes of the wealthy elite in ancient Rome functioned as both a public and a private space. A Roman male could expect his patrons and other individuals wanting his favour to gather in his atrium, he might lead a few trusted aides to a study room for work, and he might entertain important guests in his dining room. The public spaces were towards the front of the house, with the bedrooms and the family spaces towards the rear. Does this help us place the meaning of these erotic frescoes? Not really.

In the House of Caecilius a key erotic scene that is exquisitely (and presumably expensively) rendered is in a small room between the dining room and the study. In the House of the Centenary the erotic frescoes are towards the back of the house behind a dining room. In the House of the Vettii erotic pictures are on the walls of a very small room next to the kitchen. In another house an outside dining area has images of a couple making love and several ejaculating phalluses. It is a mixed picture with no seeming pattern or set rules.

Erotic frescoes, however, are not just the province of private homes, they also appear in public buildings. Unsurprisingly, the Lupanare brothel is one such place to find these images, and there are six paintings depicting sex acts between a man and a woman. There has been much scholarly debate as to whether these images equate to a menu for visitors to the brothel, but no definitive answer has yet been reached.

Sexy images in a brothel are not so surprising, sexy images at the public baths are a bit more so. The Suburban Baths, located just outside

Pompeii's walls, were more luxurious than the other public bathhouse within the city walls; its rooms were larger in size with better lighting and, in addition to the usual bathing facilities, it offered a heated swimming pool. Significantly, it had only one dressing room where both men and women would change.[4] I say 'significantly' because this is the room where we find our erotic frescoes.

Each of the eight images has a number above it and differs in what they depict from what have been found in private houses. The first two images are standard, a woman lowering herself onto her partner's penis, followed by another image of a couple in the readiness of sexual intercourse, but from then it gets odder.

The next image is a woman fellating a man, followed by a man performing oral sex on a woman, followed by an image of two women together. Next up we have a threesome, with a kneeling woman being penetrated from behind by a man, who in turn is being penetrated from behind by a man. In the next image of the series the ante is upped further with a foursome: a woman performs cunnilingus on another woman while a man fellates another man.

Now, as we've discussed earlier, both cunnilingus and men fellating men were taboo acts in ancient Rome, very much lacking in *virtus* and considered polluting and disgusting. Also, we've looked at how sex between men and boys (with some caveats) was socially acceptable, but sex between men of a similar age and standard was very much not. Finally, we've examined how the ancient Roman view of lesbianism was not terribly complimentary. All of these are depicted in the images from the Suburban Baths, so what is going on?

The answer is in the order of the images, the way they increase the level of depravity with each sex act shown until we get to that foursome. It's also in the final image that we've not yet discussed. It's not of a couple or a threesome or even a foursome, it is of a single man and its inclusion gives us an explanation; he is standing in front of a table naked, reading a scroll. The part(s) that draws the eye of the viewer are his grotesquely enlarged testicles. It's likely a metaphor for sexual frustration or built up sexual energy. Rather than partaking in the range of sex acts before him he instead prefers to read. It's a joke: the whole set of images of lovemaking are meant to be looked at (by both sexes) and laughed at.[5]

The images at the baths change how we look at that 'erotica' in the private homes of Pompeiians. If women were exposed to depictions of the most scandalous of sex acts while going for a bath, those images in the homes were unlikely to have been hidden from their eyes. Similarly, given the range of depictions of sex acts in public buildings there is no reason why house guests wouldn't have been shown the owner's latest fresco design.

Sex was not something that was hidden away, it was not secretive, it was something to be looked at or laughed at by the entire population. What is clear is the gap of perception between what we, as people living in the twenty-first century, see and what the ancient Romans saw.

We see private, sexually titillating, inappropriate pornography. The Romans saw nothing inappropriate in these images, as proven by just how many depictions there were of varied sexual positions in a multitude of different rooms. It is a fascinating peek behind the curtain of history into a world where the norms are so alien as to baffle generations of archaeologists.

The cup of mysteries

One example of this gap in our knowledge is the object discussed at the beginning of this chapter, the Warren Cup. It is more than just an image of anal sex. There are all manner of aspects to this object that raise questions that can't be answered.

We looked at the acceptable forms of same-sex relations in an earlier chapter, concluding that the proper, acceptable partner for an adult male citizen was a passive slave boy. On the Warren Cup one participant has a beard, denoting he is the elder, but his partner is not a boy, and the two are depicted as the same size. And why does the older man have a beard anyway? The cup dates to a pre-Hadrian era when Roman men did not wear beards. There are many theories surrounding the Warren Cup, and for a long time it was thought to be a forgery because of its strange images. It could be a satire on Augustan morality laws: the younger man has the hairstyle of that era, so is he perhaps meant to be a younger member of the family? Is this a commentary on the hypocrisy of Augustus and his own family's morals? Does the older man have a beard because he's a foreigner and the cup is a metaphor about the decline of Roman power, with Rome portrayed as the young man literally being buggered by the enemy?

We simply cannot know because we do not share the same cultural background and baggage. The imagery and what it means is lost to us. Possibly every single aspect of the Warren Cup, from the men to the positioning to the bed sheets, meant something to the Romans. Possibly it is simply an image of two men having sex.

Phalluses, phalluses everywhere

Mary Beard once cheerfully declared on national prime time British television, 'You can tell it's Roman because of all the willies.' We've looked so far at depictions of couples and lovemaking, but there is one image that you simply cannot escape in ancient Rome, the phallus. It is everywhere: on walls, on pavements, as décor on drinking pots, as a charm on a necklace, engraved in gemstones on rings, etched into the masonry of the Colosseum and pretty much anywhere else you can think of. What is with all the penises?

The word you will find constantly mentioned in academic papers about phallic images in Rome is apotropaic. Apotropaic means to avert evil influences and bad luck. Suddenly all those images of penises make much more sense.

One of the objects often stored in the *bulla* of young Roman boys were phallic amulets, to ward off the evil influence of any *virtus*-stealing adult. That fresco of Priapus with the huge erection on the walls of the House of Vettii is an amusing image but is there to prevent bad luck befalling the household (see image 29). The penis-shaped bell chimes with the legs of a horse found in shops were to avert bad luck on the business and the proprietor. In a world where death and destitution were a real everyday possibility everybody and every building needed a phallic protector.

Quite why and how the penis came to be thought of as a lucky charm and protection against evil is the sort of thing that keeps classicists awake at night. Perhaps it is related to the aggressive, threatening language that Romans attributed to the acts their penises would inflict on others? The penis as a powerful weapon against all manner of things? Nobody really knows. It is curiously baffling.

Curiously baffling is as good a description as any of the vast array of images of genitalia and sexual intercourse that covered all manner of surfaces in Roman society. We don't have the understanding that they did as to meanings of these images, and that makes them and Roman society all the more intriguing.

The goat man

No statue is more baffling, or more illustrative of that gap of perception then the figurine of the god Pan copulating with a goat. Who on earth would buy an image depicting bestiality, fabulous though it is?

We can partly answer this by looking at where the figure was found: the Villa of the Papyri at Herculaneum. One of the largest houses discovered there, it takes up 250m of the coastline and presented excellent sea views for its occupants. It was thought to have been once owned by Julius Caesar's father-in-law, but whoever owned it in 79 CE was both learned and educated. We know this because of how the house got its name.

It is called the Villa of Papyri because of its library. Some 1,800 scrolls, carbonised by the eruption of Vesuvius, have been discovered in total, enough to keep teams of archaeologists happily occupied trying to decipher what is written on them, while classicists keep their fingers crossed for some great lost work.

Also discovered during excavations of this villa were some truly great works of art which have now found their way to the Naples Archaeological Museum, amongst them our statue of Pan being over friendly with that goat. According to archaeological records, the Pan statue was in the garden, more precisely the south side between the portico and the pond. Also located in that same area were statues/busts of a dancer, a warrior, Pharoh Ptolomy II of Egypt, Greek poet Anacreon, an undetermined Hellenistic king, a philosopher of some sort and a bust that was once thought to be Seneca but now everyone has decided is not.

It's a mix of images that have no seeming connection, although recently the curator of antiquities at the Getty Museum in Los Angeles, Ken Lapatin, has suggested that the Pan might have been placed next to an image of the Greek poet Panyassis of Halicarnassus to create a play on words to amuse our erudite homeowner and his pals. *Pan*yassis – get it?[6]

Yes, that is a very weak gag and I like to think that our learned and moneyed occupant of the Villa of the Papyri was better than that, though perhaps not. We discussed in an earlier chapter the Sleeping Hermaphroditus and its unending appeal, and the Pan likely caused a similar affect as that statue, a state of shocked amusement. Shock at the act that is being depicted, followed by amusement as the details of the statue are taken in, most particularly the very tender, loving look Pan and his nanny goat are sharing. The guests wandering about the garden would have cracked a smile at the absurd scene presented to them. It probably created a bit of discussion over dinner. That was possibly its purpose.

Chapter 16

The Sex Life of Emperors

We have, over the course of this book, investigated what was acceptable and what was not acceptable sexual behaviour in ancient Rome. We have looked at morals and taboos, legality and illegality, and all the shades in between. No book about sex and sexuality in ancient Rome, however, would be complete though without delving into the most extreme sexual behaviour of the era, that of Rome's emperors.

The historians of the age gathered a truly extraordinarily catalogue of depravities, much of it unbelievable (because it likely never happened) on Rome's rulers. Why? Because, as we've looked at previously in this book, in Rome your private behaviour was very much seen as an indicator of your public character: the worse the bedroom behaviour, the worse the person.

Therefore, with any emperor deemed bad at their job as emperor, we find alongside their failings in the public arena a catalogue of barely believable debauchery in the private. On the reverse side, any emperor deemed good at their job will find any troublesome predilections explained away, such as this on Trajan from Cassius Dio, who after admitting that Trajan was excessively devoted to boys adds, 'In his relation with boys he harmed no one.'[1] Augustus is semi excused breaking his own adultery laws by Suetonius, 'Not even his friends could deny that he often committed adultery, though of course, they said, in justification, that he did so for reasons of state, not simple passion.'[2] Of course he did.

To end our trawl through the sex lives of the ancient Romans I've pulled out some examples of emperors whose failings in the public arena might well have been down to their exhausting private lives. Each one demonstrates clearly what the sexual taboos were in Roman society as they crash straight through them. Be warned that the following stories contain anecdotes of a truly eye-popping nature, and which will create images you'll struggle to erase from your mind. You have been warned!

Tiberius – the roaring seventies

We met Rome's second emperor earlier in the book dealing with his fanatically adulterous wife and reaping revenge for his humiliation once he succeeded her father as emperor. But Tiberius has a story of his own.

As discussed previously, Tiberius was an important member of Augustus' dynastical plans: he held important public positions, he served as a general in dangerous regimes of the empire, he was (unhappily) married off to Augustus' daughter, Julia. He was altogether suitable successor material.

Aside from that unhappy love life, being forced to divorce the woman he loved to marry a woman he didn't love, there is nothing terribly untoward in Tiberius' pre-emperor life. Yes, he's a miserable gloomy sort who had a reputation for hard drinking, but nothing whatsoever that gives any suggestion or hint that there was anything dodgy lurking beneath the taciturn exterior.

There's not a lot in his early years as emperor in Rome either. Suetonius mentions a party Tiberius attended where all the waitresses were naked, but this was apparently the hosts' usual way of serving dinner. True, he never remarries after Julia, but given how bad that marriage was, we can hardly blame him for that. We can deduce that he never got over his divorce from Vipsania, though given he was emperor it was totally within his power to insist that she divorce her husband and remarry him. He doesn't do this, and we can make whatever conclusions we like.

To read the historian Tacitus' account of Tiberius' reign to is wade through a multitude of information on regulations and trials, but very little that is salacious. This all changes when Tiberius retires to the island of Capri in 27 CE.

Tacitus tells us Tiberius departs with a few companions of senatorial rank, his favourite astrologer and some learned men. Presumably Tiberius sends for further companions since Tacitus tells us some pages later that the emperor spent his time enjoying secret orgies and having malevolent thoughts, hardly the pursuits of those learned men.

But the real juice for Tiberius' time on Capri comes from scandal-monger supreme Suetonius, who informs us that 'Some aspects of his criminal obscenity are almost too vile to discuss, much less believe.' Suetonius then helpfully lists those allegations in full so that we can judge their vile believability for ourselves.

Tiberius is said to have a fascination with erotic (and by erotic we mean filthy) images. He decorated rooms in the twelve palaces he built on Capri with indecent images, including one that reworked the mythological and unrequited love between Atalanta and Meleager.

In the myth Meleager was in love with the huntress Atalanta, but she is unwilling to marry and wishes to retain her virginity. Taking part in a boar hunt together, Meleager and Atalanta successfully killed the boar between them. However, Meleager gave Atalanta the prize since she had drawn the first blood, which enraged his uncles who couldn't accept the prize going to a mere woman.

There was an argument, and this being Greek myth, the result was a bloodbath. Meleager killed all the uncles and a couple of spectators for insulting Atlanta and was then killed himself by his own mother; an uncharacteristically low body count for mythology. Anyhow, into this tale of boar hunting and mass murder the artist of Tiberius' painting somehow manages to squeeze a scene of Atalanta performing oral sex on Meleager. The painting hung proudly in his bedroom.

As well as looking at paintings of sex, Tiberius had a living alternative in scores of attractive young boys and girls who were made to copulate in unnatural positions in front of him. To keep up the novelty Tiberius had imported certain exotically erotic books from which he would select the positions he wished to see re-enacted by his team of sex performers.

When he tired of these live sex shows he added in a role-play element by having them dress up as pan and nymphs. He had them hide in secret nooks within woods so that he could 'accidentally' come across them.

But he went far beyond these voyeuristic tendencies. During a sacrifice to the gods, the emperor took a fancy to two boys taking part in the ceremony. Immediately after the sacrifice he hurried them out of the temple and sexually assaulted them. When they complained, he had both their legs broken. A woman named Mallonia chose to commit suicide after her sexual assault by the emperor, declaring him 'that filthy mouthed hairy stinking old man.' The assault, as hinted at by the 'mouthed' in that accusation, was enforced cunnilingus.

It gets worse; the minnows were teams of small boys that were trained to swim underwater and nibble at Tiberius' genitals while the emperor enjoyed his morning swim. And if you think we really can't scrape the barrel any further on the truly depraved front, babies were allegedly employed for the purposes of fellating the emperor.

This is one hell of a catalogue of debauchery, not least because Tiberius was in his seventies by this point. Had he gone senile? Had his disappointments, both in love and life as emperor, driven him over the edge into insanity? And more to the point, where on earth did he get the stamina for all this depravity?

As we noted earlier, Tiberius' earlier sexual history is unremarkable. He passes through his adolescence, that notorious time for salacious behaviour, without a blemish to his name. Our sources would have us believe that all that time he managed to keep a lid on his unnatural desires until he got to Capri and they all burst out of him like a Pandora's box of perversion. It's not completely implausible, but alternatively it doesn't feel very likely either.

The emperor is many miles from Rome, nobody has seen him for years, access to him and Capri is heavily controlled. Even when he was in Rome Tiberius was a difficult character to read, 'besides, what Tiberius said, even when he did not aim at concealment, was – by habit or nature – always hesitant, always cryptic.'[3] Which might explain why these stories attach themselves to his name: with an unknowable emperor you can say anything about him, anything is believable.

Tiberius died, unloved, in 37 CE. The people shouted, 'To the Tiber with Tiberius!' They had a new emperor, Caligula, a golden prince who had learnt at Tiberius' knee and would come close to his adopted father in tales of perversion.

Commodus

Commodus succeeded his father, Marcus Aurelius, as emperor in 180 CE. He'd been co-emperor with his father for the previous three years and this was the first recorded instance of an emperor being born to the purple (that is, he was born when his father was already emperor). It was only the second occasion that a son succeeded his father as emperor (the first being Titus who, unlike Commodus, was an adult when his father became emperor): the previous five emperors had inherited their rule by being adopted by their predecessor as adults. They had collectively become known, by their careful management of the empire, as the 'Five Good Emperors'. Commodus brought the era of the five good emperors to an abrupt end.

Commodus should have been an excellent emperor. He'd been trained up by his father, the wise Marcus Aurelius, from childhood but it was clear from his very early days that he was grossly incapable of the role. The author of his biography in the *Historia Augusta* sets us up neatly for the depravity to come: 'For even from his earliest years he was base and dishonourable, and cruel and lewd, defiled of mouth, moreover, and debauched.'⁴ Note again, as we have throughout this book, the importance of the mouth.

Defilement of the mouth is not the only Roman cultural norm that Commodus decides to break. He is (according to our sources) a one-man taboo breaker: so much so that he was accused of being a man of a depravity by actors! Yes, those same actors who feature down the very bottom of the Roman class system, tainted by *infamia*, and who are very much not proper people to associate with. If they believed the emperor was a deviant, then he truly must have been.

Behaving lower than an actor is just one of the taboos Commodus notches up. Get your tick list ready for the rest:

1. Snogging his male partner in public. See also, 'He kept among his minions certain men named after the private parts of both sexes, and on these he liked to bestow kisses. He also had in his company a man with a male member larger than that of most animals.'⁵
2. Becoming a pimp by gathering up 300 of the most attractive women in the empire to be his personal harem. Which also broke the Lex Scantinia since some of these concubines were free women who, effectively, had been kidnapped.
3. Playing the role of the gladiator and the charioteer. Aping the *infames* and in public too!
4. Messing with clearly defined gender roles by appearing in public in women's clothes.
5. Visiting various humiliations on the senatorial class.
6. Grandiose behaviour, including renaming every single month after himself and so ignoring that humble aspect so revered in *virtus*. See also his lack of clemency, and laziness in dispatching his public duties.

Now, with Tiberius we pondered how true the stories attached to his name were and throughout this book we have queried the accuracy of our sources (looking at you, Suetonius). However, in the case of Commodus we have an actual eyewitness: the historian Cassius Dio, who was physically present during the emperor's foray into being a gladiator.

Cassius Dio records how the emperor celebrated his success in a gladiator bout with his Praetorian Prefect and secretary, 'when he had finished his sparring match, and of course won it, he would then, just as he was, kiss these companions through his helmet.'[6] Which is not quite as extreme as reported by the *Historia Augusta*, which claimed that Commodus openly snogged his male partner (but this is how massive trees of gossip sprout from small acorns).

Cassius Dio, who knew Commodus, is altogether fairer than the *Historia Augusta*. Commodus 'was not naturally wicked, but, on the contrary, as guileless as any man that ever lived.' Commodus' problem, as Cassius Dio saw it, was that he was easily led by others. This led him into, what the historian dubs 'lustful and cruel habits'.

Cassius Dio's account of the reign of Commodus is noticeably lacking in sexploits. There is no mention of the free woman brothel for instance, or any of the other defilements mentioned by the *Historia Augusta*. Which sadly means the tales are likely to be invented, or at the very least exaggerated beyond any semblance of truth.

What we get in Cassius Dio is the grandiosity and delusions of an emperor: the gold statue of himself he ordered, the renaming of every single month after himself, the titles he insisted the Senate address him by: 'The Emperor Caesar Lucius Aelius Aurelius Commodus Augustus Pius Felix Sarmaticus Germanicus Maximus Britannicus, Pacifier of the Whole Earth, Invincible, the Roman Hercules, Pontifex Maximus, Holder of the Tribunician Authority for the eighteenth time, Imperator for the eighth time, Consul for the seventh time, Father of his Country, to consuls, praetors, tribunes, and the fortunate Commodian Senate, greeting.'

The Commodus of Cassius Dio greets his senators at the amphitheatre in a silk tunic interwoven with gold, then nips in to change into a purple robe with gold spangles which he accessorises with an Indian crown of many gems. Cassius Dio's Commodus is a mixture of the absurd and the terrifying, and nowhere is this more apparent than in the greatest anecdote ever recorded in all Roman history. Greatest because it's all true and it reveals exactly what it is like to have to serve an emperor who has entirely lost the plot.

Cassius Dio and his fellow senators had been summoned to the amphitheatre to watch the emperor pretend to be a gladiator, an event that took place over fourteen days. The emperor was keen to show off how brilliantly he could murder wildlife. Cassius Dio helpfully records the tally of creatures that Commodus despatched, which included tigers, hippos and elephants. On one particular day during this orgy of violence Cassius Dio tells us:

> Having killed an ostrich and cut off his head, he came up to where we were sitting, holding the head in his left hand and in his right hand raising aloft his bloody sword; and though he spoke not a word, yet he wagged his head with a grin, indicating that he would treat us in the same way. And many would indeed have perished by the sword on the spot, for laughing at him (for it was laughter rather than indignation that overcame us), if I had not chewed some laurel leaves, which I got from my garland, myself, and persuaded the others who were sitting near me to do the same.[7]

This sums up Commodus' character entirely: laughable but not a man to laugh at. He was eventually assassinated, after several previous attempts had failed, by his mistress, Marcia, who served him up a plate of poisoned beef. When the emperor threw that back up, a wrestler named (ironically) Narcissus was sent in to strangle him.

Elagabalus

Varius Avitus Bassianus became emperor at the age of fourteen in 218 CE, at which point he acquired a shiny new name, Marcus Aurelius Antonius. Neither name sticks to him and to history he will be known as Elagabalus, after the sun god for which he once served as head priest.

Elagabalus ruled as emperor for only four years, nowhere near as long as Commodus or Tiberius, but the sheer amount of depravity, debauchery, decadence and dodginess he manages to squeeze into those four years is impressive. It was handy that it was his mother, Julia Soaemias, and his grandmother, Julia Maesa, who did all the actual ruling bits, such as attending the senate, so that he could fit in all the debauchery.

What was he up to? Over to Cassius Dio, 'He used his body both for doing and allowing many strange things, which no one could endure to tell or hear of; but his most conspicuous acts, which it would be impossible to conceal, were the following.'[8]

Elagabalus is the epitome of the effeminate male we looked at in a previous chapter. Cassius Dio says he more or less had the appearance of a man, but he gave himself away by his actions and his voice. One such giveaway is the way Elagabalus moves, 'He used to dance, not only in the orchestra, but also, in a way, even while walking, performing sacrifices, receiving salutations, or delivering a speech.'[9] This raises a lot of questions: is the emperor a fidgety teenager? Or is he feeling the power of dance course through his body?

Elagabalus is the ultimate in effeminacy: not only does he remove all his body hair, he also wears make up and a hairnet and heads down to the local taverns in a woman's wig. He is a passive homosexual partner, acquiring a series of husbands and calls himself their wife or mistress. An obsession with large penises sees his hire agents scouring the empire for men to add to his collection and he opens a public bath in the hope of acquiring some more well-endowed specimens. And finally, just in case you had any doubts on the subject of Elagabalus' masculinity, 'He carried his lewdness to such a point that he asked the physicians to contrive a woman's vagina in his body by means of an incision, promising them large sums for doing so.'[10]

Some of these tales, I think we can state clearly, are invented. This is borne out by the inclusion of human sacrifice amongst Elagabalus' many alleged crimes, which always reeks of trying to slander with the worst possible thing you can think of (such as in the Bacchanalia scandal we discussed in an earlier chapter). Unsurprisingly, Elagabalus is also accused of torturing and sacrificing children. So, what are we to make of Elagabalus? Amongst all these strange tales is a recurrent theme, play.

Take this story from Cassius Dio, 'He set aside a room in the palace and there committed his indecencies, always standing nude at the door of the room, as the harlots do, and shaking the curtain which hung from gold rings, while in a soft and melting voice he solicited the passers-by.

There were, of course, men who had been specially instructed to play their part.'[11]

His trips to the local taverns include him playing at being a prostitute. He would ride his chariot at the palace with the imperial freedmen, equestrians and senators as his audience. Alongside wearing make-up, we are told he also worked wool, just as women did, and then there were those marriages to his husbands. He's playing a series of roles using his position as emperor to manufacture the desired scenarios. Elagabalus is not unlike Nero who similarly created his own reality as an artist and appears to have been fond of sexual role play.

I think what we must remember is that he is only a teenager when he becomes emperor and clearly not a very mature one. Nero, similarly, was seventeen when he became emperor, and look how that turned out. Given unlimited license to do whatever he wished, Elagabalus explored his sexuality, his masculinity and his identity, leaving the politics to his female relatives. This was never going to go down well in Rome, and it didn't. The aggressively male Roman state reached the limit of its tolerance on Elagabalus' effeminate antics. He was murdered in a palace coup aged only eighteen.

Author's Note

I hope you have enjoyed this speedy trip around sex and sexuality in ancient Rome. As it's a single volume it would have been impossible to cover every aspect of a subject that is so detailed, complex, varied and rich, such as the Christian experience in Rome for instance. Unfortunately, there was simply not the space to give an airing to every theory and paper on Roman sex. Also, be aware that the scholarship and thinking on this subject is fast moving. But I hope I have delivered a basic background on how the Romans viewed, thought and talked about the subject.

For further reading check out the bibliography. Or even better, plan a trip to the nearest museum that has a copy of the Sleeping Hermaphroditus. I promise you it'll make you smile.

L.J. Trafford September 2020

Notes

Chapter 1: Language
1. Catullus, poem 16.
2. Catullus, poem 21.
3. Catullus, poem 37.
4. Most likely born of the imagination of the likes of Juvenal, who speculate and expand upon the humiliation a wronged husband might inflict on his wife's lover, including castration.
5. The jury is out on whether Catullus is using obscenity in a clever and poetic way or whether he's just really wound up and expressing his thoughts as they are. There are many commentaries and essays written on the use of foul language in Catullus which make for entertaining reading and are a useful insight into what Classics professors do all day.
6. Appian, *The Civil Wars* 5.3.19, who says of Fulvia that she was 'moved by a women's jealousy'.
7. Modern-day Perugia in the Italian region of Umbria.
8. Martial, *Epigrams*, 11.20.
9. Much of the non-obscene graffiti quotes from literature, such as Virgil's *Aeneid*. The sheer amount of written material found at Pompeii from graffiti to legal documents to the labels on jars suggest most of the inhabitants had some form of reading ability. Mary Beard's *Pompeii, Life of a town* discusses this in some detail, p184.
10. In 47 CE.
11. Tacitus, *Annals* 11.2.
12. Plutarch, *Life of Pompey*, 48.
13. But also because of the increasing political violence on the street.
14. Plutarch, *Julius Caesar*, 4.
15. Martial , *Epigrams*, 1.42.
16. Cicero, *Pro Caelio*, 48.
17. Plutarch, *Life of Mark Antony*, 10.
18. Tacitus, *Annals*, 4.4.3

Chapter 2: Controlling Desire: A Brief History of Morality Laws
1. Tacitus, *Germania*, 19.
2. Livy, *The History of Rome*.
3. Plutarch, *Life of Aemilius Paulus*.
4. Seneca, letters, 114.9.
5. Plutarch, *Life of Cato the Elder*, 16.5
6. Juvenal, *Satire*, 6.88.
7. Livy, *History of Rome*, 34.3.
8. The rostra was a speaking platform in the Forum. It is the location of all manner of exciting historical events, such as Mark Antony's famous speech to Romans after the assassination of Julius Caesar.

9. Plutarch, *Life of Cato the Elder*, 19.3.
10. Martial, *Epigrams*, 10.8.

Chapter 3: Ideals: The Virtuous Man

1. Galen, *The affections and errors of the soul*, 10.55–56.
2. The Ligurians were based in North West Italy.
3. Plutarch, *Life of Aemilius Paullus*, 39.8.
4. Ibid, 5.4.
5. The US city of Cincinnati is named after him.
6. Livy, 3.26.
7. Columella, *De Re Rustica*, Preface, 1.17.
8. Ibid, 1.8.15.
9. Horace, *Ars*, 161–5.
10. Cicero, *Pro Caelio*, 42.
11. Cicero, speech against Catiline 2.23.
12. Plautus, *Curculio*.

Chapter 4: Ideals: The Chaste Woman

1. That there are numerous amendments to this law shows that there was very real concern over its application and potential misuse.
2. For those who don't know, Oedipus famously unwittingly killed his birth father and married his birth mother. His discovery of which is the subject of a Sophocles play.
3. Juvenal, *Satire*, 6.
4. Soranus, *Gynaecology*, 2.10.79.
5. Artemidorus, *The Interpretation of Dreams*, 1.15.
6. Oxyrhynchus Papyri 744.
7. Though this was ended under the emperor Antoninus Pius, 131 –161 CE.
8. Soranus, *Gynaecology*, 9.34.
9. Marcianus, *Institutes*, Book 10. 7.
10. CIL 1.2.1221 (ILS 7472) & CIL 1.01221 = CIL 6.9499 (ILS 7472)
11. Livy, *History of Rome*, 1.58.
12. A decemvir was an important post in the Roman Republic. There were ten of them, hence the name.
13. Livy, *History of Rome*, 3.45.7.
14. Ibid, 3.45.11.
15. 218–201 BCE.
16. Ancient battle loss numbers are notoriously inaccurate, sources claiming here that 50,000 Romans were killed, which is almost certainly an exaggeration. But whatever the figure it was a great humiliation for Rome and they never forgot it.
17. The Sibylline Oracle was a collection of books that claimed to list the predictions of a famous oracle. They were consulted at times of national crisis, such as this one.
18. Ovid, *Fasti*, 4.319.
19. Amphitheatres were seated by rank with senators at the front, equestrians behind, then free men, then right at the back women and slaves.
20. Pliny the Younger, letters 43.
21. *Historia Augusta*, Life of Elagbalus, 6.6.
22. *Pliny the Younger*, 6.24.
23. Arrias' story features in letter 16 in Book 3 of Pliny's letters.
24. Roman punishments are gratuitously unfair. Whereas an ordinary citizen might find themselves in the arena, the elite will be sent a letter telling them to commit suicide or else.

25. It should be noted that this 'home' belonged to one Milo who had been exiled. In his exile Turia's husband had purchased the property. The gang that Turia fights off were Milo's men. He is understandably a bit upset his house has been sold to someone else against his will.
26. Although Suetonius, our gossip-master on emperors, did write a series of biographies called *On Famous Whores*. Tragically, this book got lost somewhere between antiquity and now.
27. Suetonius, *Life of Augustus*, 73.1.
28. Tacitus, *Histories*, 1.73.
29. Several prominent members of Nero's court were targeted both by Galba and by vigilantes. That Calvia escapes this despite the clamours for retribution is testament to her political wiliness.
30. Tacitus, *Histories*, 1.73.
31. Juvenal, *Satire*, 6.1.

Chapter 5: Neither Male nor Female
 1. Pliny the Elder, *Natural Histories*, Book 7,33.
 2. All the stories about sex changes are in Pliny the Elder, *Natural Histories*, Book 7.
 3. Pliny the Elder, *Natural Histories*, Book 7,36.
 4. From an account of the Epitome of medicine compiled in the seventh century.
 5. *Historia Augusta*, Life of Alexander Severus, 23.4.
 6. Ammianus Marcellinus, 14.11.
 7. Paezon was sold by Sejanus for an astonishing 50 million sesterces.
 8. Statius, *Silvae*, 3.4.
 9. Virgil, *Aeneid*, 1.12.
 10. Martial writes several begging poems to Domitian's secretary, Parthenius, asking him to pass his poems onto the emperor.
 11. A Phrygian cap is not dissimilar to a Smurf's hat. It was known in Rome as the liberty cap since it was worn by freedmen.
 12. Ovid, *Fasti*, 4.4.
 13. Ulpianus, on duties of the pro consul book 7.
 14. Book 3, 4a, *Opinions of Paulus*.

Chapter 6: How to be Sexy: Beauty and Fashion
 1. Ovid on Cosmetics.
 2. Ovid, *The Art of Love*, 3.3.
 3. Although it's not nearly as miraculous as cabbage, which the Romans have as a cure for everything from headaches to sprains to fistulas to preventing wine induced intoxication. It's also good for eyesight too.
 4. Juvenal, *Satire*, 6.
 5. Pliny the Elder, *Natural Histories*, Book 13, 20.
 6. The produce of the sea that Pliny is finding particularly decaying is the purple dye that was made from crushing sea snails.
 7. Martial, *Epigrams*, 3.55.
 8. Check out historical hair investigator Janet Stephens on YouTube, who makes some worthy attempts at recreating these styles, including the Flavian lady hair-do.
 9. Martial, *Epigrams*, 3.43.
 10. Ovid, *Art of Love*, 1.39.
 11. According to the brilliant ORBIs website from Stanford University, which calculates the time it takes to travel pretty much anywhere in the ancient world.
 12. Ovid, *Art of Love*, 3.4.
 13. Martial, *Epigrams*, 10.90.
 14. Pliny the Elder. *Natural Histories*, 29, 26.
 15. Martial, *Epigrams*, 9.27.
 16. Suetonius, *Life of Otho*.

17. Cicero, letters to Atticus, 1.14.
18. Pliny the Elder, *Natural Histories*, 11, 78.
19. Horace, *Satires*, 1.2.
20. In modern-day Lebanon.
21. Ovid, *Art of Love*, 2.4.
22. Martial, *Epigrams*, 11.100.
23. Ibid, 10.47.
24. Horace, *Satires*, 1.2.
25. Although if a Jew circumcised his slave who was not Jewish they faced deportation or death.
26. *The Priapeia*, 12.
27. Ibid, 27.
28. Ibid, 25.
29. Seneca, *Natural Questions*, 1.16.
30. Martial, *Epigrams*, 9.60.
31. *Historia Augusta*, Life of Elagabalus, 5.3
32. Aristophanes, *Clouds*.
33. If you really want to read the full poem it is Book 11.21. Although it is extremely hard to find in an English translation, clearly because it's so nasty no one wanted to translate it. You have been warned. Of course as a satirist Martial is being deliberately shocking and provocative.
34. Martial, *Epigrams*, 7.18.

Chapter 7: Finding Love: Courting on the Streets of Rome

1. Plautus, *Curculio*.
2. Tibullus, 1.2.
3. Ibid, 1.2.
4. Propertius, 1.16.
5. Ovid, *Art of Love*, 1.6.
6. Horace, *Satires*, 1.2.
7. I'm being unfair to Ovid. He also wrote two epic works, the *Fasti* and *Metamorphoses*, which are both acclaimed.
8. Rather confusingly since sources seem clear that women were seated separate to men at the games. Either the seating demarcation wasn't as strict as we've been led to believe or Ovid is making this entire episode up.
9. Ovid, *Art of Love*, Book 1.7.
10. Juvenal, *Satire*, 6.
11. Seneca, letters, 51.
12. Penelope being the steadfast loyal wife to Odysseus. Helen being the faithless wife whose faithlessness started off the Trojan War.
13. Suetonius, *Life of Augustus*, 69.1
14. *Historia Augusta*, Life of Lucius Verus, 5.2.
15. Horrifyingly, slaves were the persistent victims of sexual abuse at the hands of their masters.

Chapter 8: Getting Down to Business: Sex

1. Pliny the Elder, *Natural Histories*, 10.171.
2. Soranus, *Gynaecology*, 1.7.
3. He claims that the wives of Brutus, Pompey and the Gracchi were fully up for it – without any evidence to back that up.
4. Ovid, *Art of Love*, 2.19.
5. Ovid has an alternative version where Tiresias, rather than leave the snakes be, beats them again with a stick, showing he/she had learnt absolutely nothing.
6. Artemidorus, *The Interpretation of Dreams*, 1.79.

7. You will be entirely unsurprised to learn that Sigmund Freud was familiar with Artemidorus' work.
8. Artemidorus, *The Interpretation of Dreams* , 1.78.6.
9. Ibid, 4.59.

Chapter 9: Sexual Problems and Solutions
1. Galen, *Mixtures*, 2.4.
2. Ovid, *Art of Love*, 3.7.
3. Artemidorus, *Interpretation of Dreams*, 1.45.
4. Horace, *Epode*, 12.
5. Pliny the Elder, *Natural Histories*, 30.49.
6. Soranus, *Gynaecology*, 3.29.
7. Ibid, 4.26.
8. Hippocrates, *The Seed & The Nature of the Child*, 13.
9. Tertullian, *De Anima*, 25.
10. Ovid, *Art of Love*, 2.14.
11. The rumoured father being her uncle, Domitian, which is probably nonsense.
12. Soranus, *Gynaecology*, 1.35.
13. Celsus, *On Medicine* 4.28.
14. Mentioned in chapter 4.

Chapter 10: Love Hurts: When Love Goes Wrong
1. A potted selection of complaints from Propertius' *Elegies*.
2. Poor Propertius appears constantly on edge, fearing Cynthia's temper.
3. See 4.8 where she physically attacks poor hapless Propertius *'to strike my face with perverse hands, put her mark on my neck, drew blood with her mouth, and most of all struck my eyes that deserved.'*
4. Plutarch, *Life of Lucullus*, 34.
5. Ibid, 38.
6. Caesar would later divorce Pompeia with the justification that 'Caesar's wife must be above suspicion.'
7. Catullus, 79.
8. Letters to Atticus. 1.18.
9. Catullus, 87.
10. Catullus, 85.
11. Catullus, 70.
12. Catullus, 32.

Chapter 11: Managing Affairs of the Heart: Religion and Magic
1. Found at Bath, UK.
2. ILS 8753, quoted in *As The Romans Did*, Jo-Ann Shelton.
3. Found in a field in Baldock, Hertfordshire.
4. Other groups of individuals who repeatedly get removed from Rome for causing trouble include Jews, philosophers and ballet dancers.
5. Pliny is similarly sceptical about the gods and life after death, it should be noted.
6. Ovid, *Art of Love*, 3.6.
7. Artemidorus, *The Interpretation of Dreams*, 1.78.
8. Plautus, 'Miles Glorianus', line 691.
9. Martial, *Epigrams*, 7.54.
10. Juvenal, *Satire*, 6.
11. Lex Cornelia quoted in the Opinions of Paulus, 5.23.14.

12. Propertius, *Elegies*, Book 3.6.
13. Ibid.
14. The Magic Papryi, PGM 61.
15. Ibid, PGM 4 296.
16. Tibullus, *Elegies*, 1.2.
17. Ibid.
18. Horace, *Epode*, 5.
19. Juvenal, *Satire*, 6.
20. Quoted from Robert Knapp, *Invisible Romans*, p14.
21. Found in Egypt and dated to the third or fourth century CE. 'When Spells work magic' by Christopher A. Farone, quoted in the journal *Archaeology*, Vol. 56, No. 2, March/April 2003.
22. Ibid.
23. *Sentences of Paulus* 5.23.15–18.
24. Apuleius, *The Defence*.
25. Ovid, *Fasti* 4.
26. Livy, *History of Rome*, Book 39.
27. Ibid.

Chapter 12: Adultery
1. Horace, *Satires*, 1.2.
2. Mary Beard, *SPQR*, p316.
3. Cassius Dio, 54.16.
4. It probably didn't help that he dumped his wife, Octavia, who happened to be the sister of Octavian/Augustus, to take up with Cleopatra.
5. Cicero, *Pro Caelio*, 35.
6. Public positions in Rome had minimum age requirements. To stand for quaestor you had to be at least thirty, for the highest position of consul forty-two was the minimum age. Augustus completely ignored these age-old rules, granting stepson Drusus the right to assume any public role five years earlier and appointing his grandsons, Gaius and Lucius, designated consuls at the age of only twenty.
7. Suetonius, *Life of Augustus*, 64.
8. Including some top-quality aqueducts and functioning sewers. As well as every battle that Augustus ever took part in, or rather didn't because he had Agrippa to do that sort of thing for him.
9. Suetonius, *Life of Tiberius*, 68.
10. Macrobius, *Saturnalia*, 2.5.
11. Ibid.
12. Romans have a very strange habit of giving their daughters all the same name. For instance, Mark Antony had two daughters, both called Antonia. Sometimes Minor or Major were used to distinguish, but that only worked in a household of two daughters.
13. One is kind of reminded of discussions re Madonna's use of outrage in the 90s when TV commentators discussed that the only thing left for her to do that would shock the public was having a child, which she did shortly afterwards.
14. Papinianus, *On Adultery*, Book 2.
15. Ulpianus, *On Adultery*, Book 8.
16. Papinianus, *On Adultery*, Book 2.
17. Papinianus. *On Adultery*, Book 2.
18. Zosimus, 2.29.2.
19. Zonarus, *Epitome*, 13.2.

Chapter 13: Homosexuality
1. Gellius, 6.12, quoted in Richlin, Amy, *The Garden of Priapus*.
2. Seneca, letters 114.6.
3. Suetonius, *Life of Caligula, 52*.
4. Juvenal, *Satire*, 2.1.
5. Cicero, *Against Piso*, 11.25.
6. Juvenal, *Satire*, 2.2.
7. Martial, *Epigrams*, 7.58.
8. Juvenal, *Satire*, 6.
9. Suetonius, *Life of Caligula,36*
10. Seneca, *Controversies*, 4.
11. Petronius, *Satyricon*, 75.
12. Horace, *Satires*, 1.2.
13. The Opinions of Julius Paulus, Book 2.32.
14. Suetonius, *Life of Nero*, 29.
15. Tacitus, *Annals*, 15.37.
16. Suetonius, *Life of Nero*, 29.
17. Suetonius, *Life of Vitellius*, 12.
18. Tacitus, *Histories*, 2.57.
19. Catullus, 48.
20. Catullus, 99.
21. Tibullus, 1.4.
22. Marital, *Epigrams*, 12.75.
23. Seneca, Letters 47.7.
24. Pausianias, *Tour of Greece*, 8.9.9.
25. *Historia Augusta*, Life of Hadrian.
26. Martial, *Epigrams*, 10.8.
27. *Historia Augusta*, Life of Alexander Severus, 24.
28. Canon 12.
29. Theodosian Code 9.7.3.
30. Juvenal, *Satire*, 6.
31. Martial, *Epigrams*, 1.90.
32. Martial, *Epigrams*, 7.70.
33. Lucian, *Amores*, 28.
34. PSI 1.28 12ff.

Chapter 14: Undesirable Partners
1. Rules of Ulpianus 13.
2. Suetonius, *Life of Otho*. 2.
3. Ulpianus, on the Lex Julia, Book 2.
4. Antonia is one of those imperial women who was connected to everyone. She was Augustus' niece, Tiberius' sister-in-law, Caligula's grandmother and Nero's great grandmother.
5. There is absolutely no evidence for this. It is entirely speculation.
6. Cassius Dio, Book 65.14.
7. Cassius Dio, Book 61.7.
8. Plutarch, *Life of Pompey*, 2.
9. Plutarch, *Life of Lucullus*, 6.
10. Plutarch, *Life of Galba*, 14.
11. Discussed at some length in Mary Beard's book, *Pompeii*.
12. Artemidorus, *The Interpretation of Dreams*, 1.78.3.
13. Ulpianus, 'On the Edict', in *Digest* 23.43.

14. Martial, *Epigrams*, 9.2.
15. The Emperors Theodosius, Arcadius, and Honorius to Rufinus, Praetorian Prefect.
16. Juvenal, *Satire*, 6.
17. Letters to Atticus, 10.10.
18. 477 (F 9, 26) Cicero to Paetus.
19. Suetonius, *Life of Caligula*, 55.
20. Ibid.
21. Martial, *Epigrams*, 11.13.
22. Suetonius, *Life of Tiberius*, 37.
23. Suetonius, *Life of Nero*, 26.
24. Petronius, *Satyricon*, 52.
25. Juvenal, *Satire*, 6.
26. Tacitus, Annals 14.
27. Cicero, *Pro Caelio*, 32.
28. Ibid.
29. Cassius Dio, 46.18.
30. Suetonius, *Life of Claudius*, 30.
31. Juvenal, *Satire*, 2.1.
32. Paulus on Sabinus, Book 4.
33. Papinianus, Questions, 32.
34. Artemidorus, 1.78.8.
35. Apuleius, *The Golden Ass*, Book 10.
36. Juvenal, *Satire*, 6.
37. Seneca letters.
38. Martial, *On Spectacles*, 5.

Chapter 15: Sexual Imagery

1. The celebrated Meroe head (which will forever be to me Scary Augustus head), his eyes don't so much as follow you round the room but curse you from every corner of it.
2. Pliny the Elder, *Natural Histories*, 36.4.
3. The reason for Ovid's exile remains murky and theories abound as to whether he was involved with the scandal of Augustus' daughter, Julia, or whether it was that his *Art of Love* did not chime with the era. Or possibly because he created a load of sex pests at the circus.
4. There is an ongoing, unresolved debate as to whether the Romans had special times for women to bath or days. Or whether there was mixed bathing.
5. See John R. Clarke's *Looking at love making* for a full discussion of these images.
6. As discussed in Mary Beard's column, 'A Don's Life' in *TES*.

Chapter 16: The Sex life of Emperors

1. Cassius Dio, 68.6.
2. Suetonius, *Life of Augustus*, 69.
3. Tacitus, *Annals*, 1.9.
4. *Historia Augusta*, Life of Commodus, 1.7.
5. *Historia Augusta*, Life of Commodus, 10.
6. Cassius Dio, 73.19.
7. Ibid, 73.21.
8. Ibid, 80.13.
9. Ibid, 79.14.
10. Ibid, 79.16.7.
11. Ibid, 69.13.

Bibliography

The Penguin Dictionary of Classical Mythology, (edited by Stephen Kershaw) (Penguin Books: 1991).

Apuleius, Lucius, *The Golden Ass, (translated by Robert Graves)*, (Penguin Classics: 1990).

Artemidorus, *The Interpretation of Dreams (translated by Martin Hammond)*, (Oxford World's Classics: 2020).

Beard, Mary, *SPQR: A History of Ancient Rome*, (Profile Books: 2016).

Beard, Mary, *Pompeii: The Life of a Roman Town*, (Profile Books: 2008).

Birley, Anthony R., *Hadrian, the restless Emperor*, (Routledge: 2000).

Catullus, *The Shorter Poems (translated by John Godwin)*, (Oxbrow Books: 2007).

Clarke, John R, *Looking at Love Making; Constructions of Sexuality in Roman Art*, (University of California Press: 2001).

Chrystal, Paul, *In Bed with the Romans*, (Amberley: 2017).

Columella, *De Re Rustica*.

Danziger, Danny and Purcell, Nicholas, *Hadrian's Empire*, (Hodder and Stoughton: 2005).

Dickie, Matthew, *Magic and Magicians in The Graeco Roman World*, (Routledge: 2001).

Dunn, Daisy, *Catullus' Bedspread*, (William Collins: 2017).

Dupont, Florence, *Daily Life in Ancient Rome*, (Blackwell: 1992).

Edwards, Catherine, *The Politics of Immorality in Ancient Rome*, (Cambridge University Press: 1993).

Galen, *Selected Works (translated by P.N. Singer)*, (Oxford University Press: 1997).

Goldhill, Simon, *Love, Sex & Tragedy; Why Classics Matters*, (John Murray: 2004).

Graf, Fritz, *Magic in the Ancient World*, (Harvard: 1997).

Hallett, Judith P and Skinner, Marilyn B, editors, *Roman Sexualities*, (Princeton University Press: 1977).

Hippocratic Writings, *(translated by Professor Geoffrey Earnest Richard Lloyd)* (Penguin Books: 1983).

Historia Augusta, Lives of the Later Caesars (translated by Anthony Birley), (Penguin Classics: 1976).

Horace, *Epodes (translated by A.S.Kline)* 2005.

Justinian, *The Code of Justinian, (translated by Samuel P Scott)*, (Cincinnati, 1932).

Juvenal, *The Sixteen Satires (translated by Peter Green)*, (Penguin Books: 2004).

Knapp, Robert, *Invisible Romans*, (Profile: 2013).

Laes, Christian and Johann Strubbe, *Youth in the Roman Empire: The Young and Restless Years*, (CUU: 2014).

Livy, *The Early History of Rome, (translated by Aubrey De Selincourt)*, (Penguin Classics: 1971).

Livy, *Rome and the Mediterranean (translated by Henry Bettenson)*, (Penguin Books: 1976).

Maranon, Gregorio, *Tiberius – A study in resentment*, (Hollis and Carter: 1956).

Marcellinus, Ammianus, *The Later Roman Empire (translated by Walter Hamilton)*, (Penguin Classics: 1986).

Martial, *The Epigrams* (translated by James Michie), (Penguin Books: 1978).

Masterson, Mark, *Man to Man; Desire, Homosexuality and Authority in Late Roman Manhood*, (Ohio State University Press: 2014).

McGinn, A.J. Prostitution, *Sexuality and the law in ancient Rome*, (Oxford University Press: 1998).

Mohr, Melissa, *Holy Shit – A Brief History of Swearing*, (Oxford University Press: 2013).

Ovid, *Fasti (Translated by A.J.Boyle and R.D.Woodard)*, (Penguin Books: 2004).

Ovid, *The Love Poems* (Translated by *A.D.Melville*), (Oxford World's Classics: 2008).

Pausanias, *Guide to Greece, (translated by Peter Levi)*, (Penguin Classics: 1971).

Petronius, *The Satyricon, (translated by P.G. Walsh)*, (Oxford World's Classics: 2009).

Pliny the Elder, *Natural History: A Selection (translated by John Healey)*, (Penguin Books: 1991).

Pliny, *The Letters of the Younger Pliny (translated by Betty Radice)*, (Penguin Books: 1969).

Plutarch, *Roman Lives (translated by Robin Waterfield)*, (Oxford World's Classics: 1999).

Pomeroy, Sarah B, *Goddesses Whores, Wives and Slaves: Women in Classical Antiquity*, (Pimlico: 1994).

Richlin, Amy, *The Garden of Priapus*, (Oxford University Press: 1992).

Roberts, Paul, *Life and death in Pompeii and Herculaneum*, (British Museum Press; 2013).

Seneca, *Letters from a Stoic (translated by Robin Campbell)*, (Penguin Books: 2004).

Shelton, Jo-Ann, *As the Romans Did: A Sourcebook in Roman Social History*, (Oxford University Press: 1988).

Smith, R.R.R, *Antinous: boy made god*, (Ashmolean: 2018).

Southern, Emma, *Agrippina: Empress, Exile, Hustler, Whore*, (Unbound: 2018).

Soranus, *Gynaecology*, (Baltimore John Hopkins Press: 1956).

Southern, Pat, *Domitian: Tragic Tyrant*, (Routledge: 1997).

Statius, *Complete Works*, (Delphi Classics: 2014).

Suetonius, *The Twelve Caesars (translated by Robert Graves)*, (Penguin Books: 1989).

Tacitus, *The Annals of Imperial Rome* (translated by Michael Grant, (Penguin Books: 1989).

Tacitus, *The Histories (translated by Kenneth Wellesley)*, (Penguin Books: 1995).

Toner, Jerry, *How to Manage your Slaves*, (Profile Books: 2015).

Toner, Jerry, *Popular Culture in Ancient Rome*, (Polity Press: 2009).

Tougher, Shaun, *The Eunuch in Byzantine History and Society*, (Routledge: 2008).

Turcan, Robert, *The Cults of the Roman Empire*, (Blackwell: 1996).

Williams, Craig A, *Roman Homosexuality*, (Oxford University Press: 1999).

Index